D1193889

Understanding Sexual Medicine

Other books by Ivor Felstein:

Later Life
Sex and the Longer Life
A Change of Face and Figure
Snakes and Ladders
The Medical Shorthand Typist (co-author)
Looking at Retirement
Living to be a Hundred
Sexual Pollution
Sex in Later Life

Chapters in:

BMA Book of Executive Health
Visual Dictionary of Sex
Well-Being
Sexuality in Later Years
Book of Life
Mind Alive
Doctors' Knowledge
La Sexualité du Troisieme Age

Understanding Sexual Medicine

A Guide for Family Practitioners and Students

By

Ivor Felstein

Senior Physician and Psychotherapist
Bolton and Manchester, UK

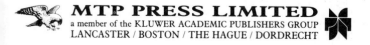

MTP PRESS LIMITED
a member of the KLUWER ACADEMIC PUBLISHERS GROUP
LANCASTER / BOSTON / THE HAGUE / DORDRECHT

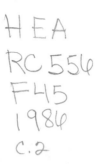
Published in UK and Europe by
MTP Press Limited
Falcon House
Lancaster, England

British Library Cataloguing in Publication Data

Felstein, Ivor
    Understanding sexual medicine.
    1. Sexual disorders
    I. Title
    616.6'9   RC556

    ISBN 0-85200-982-8

Published in the USA by
MTP Press
A division of Kluwer Academic Publishers
101 Philip Drive
Norwell, MA 02061, USA

Library of Congress Cataloging-in-Publication Data

Felstein, Ivor, 1933-
    Understanding sexual medicine.

    Bibiography:p.
    Includes index.
    1. Sexual disorders. 2. Psychosexual disorders.
    3. Sex therapy. I. Title.
    [DNLM: 1. Phychosexual Disorders.
    2. Sex Behavior. 3. Sex Disorders. WM 611 F214u]
    RC556.F45 1986   616.85'83   86-20015
    ISBN 0-85200-982-8

Typeset by Bycomp Limited, Farnham, Surrey
Printed and bound by Butler & Tanner Limited, Frome and London

Contents

1 Nature of human sexuality - and GP counselling
Aims of this book   1
What is sexuality ?   2
The significance of male sex hormone   4
Contributors to sexual drive   5
The GP as counsellor   7

2 Expressing our sexuality - and patterns of sexual drive
Common forms of sexual expression   11
Other forms of sexual expression   14
Patterns of sexual drive   17
Changed expectations   18
Effects of illness and drugs   19
Video culture   20
Environment - and obesity   20

3 Coitus in view today
Current view of coitus   23
Physiological variations   27
Coital positions   27
Some controversial points   30
Surrrogates   31
Physiological puzzles   31

4 Common sexual problems in the male partner
Erectile dysfunction   36
Ejaculatory dysfunction   45
Altered libido   49
Anxiety effects   50
Deviations and difficulties   53
Organic illness   62

Mental illness	71
Drugs	73

5 Common sexual problems in the female partner

Altered libido	79
Non-sexual marital pathologies	82
Violence and aggression	83
Dyspareunia	84
Pregnancy	86
Infection	86
Performance anxieties	87
Cosmetic turn-offs	89
Religion	90
Pregnancy - again	91
Menopause and PMT	92
Vaginismus	93
Organic discomforts	94
Drugs - again	95
Alcohol	96
The pill	96
Physical illnesses	97
Chronic diseases	97
Surgery effects	99

6 Disability, handicap and sexuality

Handicap and disability	101
Type of problems	102
An approach	104

7 Therapies and counselling

Therapeutic approaches to sexual dysfunction	107
Patterns of presenting problems	108
History taking	109
The clinical examination	111
Diagnosis and prognosis	112
Styles of therapy	115
Partner types	116
Other approaches to sex counselling and therapy	116
Barriers	118
Mixed therapy approach	119
The limitation and therapy	119
A fuller history	120

Adaptable techniques 121
Therapy of common sexual problems 123
Reduced or absent libido 123
Erectile dysfunction - emotional or psycho-
      logical blocking 125
Circumcision 128
Phobias - and organic disorders 129
Therapy of female partner problems 130
Hormone replacement therapy 130
Vaginismus 131
Dyspareunia 132
Sex drive stimulation 134
Encouraging orgasm 134
Performance anxiety 136
Cosmetic surgery 136
Sexual activity after an acute illness 137
Headache and sexual function 138
Honeymoon cystitis and the urethral syndrome 138
Medical therapy for erection 139
Surgical therapy for male dysfunction 140
'Stuffing' as therapy 141
Criteria of success in sex therapy 142
Sex after sixty 142

Selected bibliography 145

Index
Index of Persons 147
Index of Subjects 149

ACKNOWLEDGEMENT

Illustrations devised and prepared by:

MRS E. GOSLING

Medical photographer*

and

MR A. JACKSON

Senior medical photographer*

(* Currently of Dept. of Medical Illustration,
Bolton General Hospital, Lancs)

1
Nature of Human Sexuality - and GP Counselling

AIMS OF THIS BOOK

Sexual behaviour is a significant part of total human behaviour. In clinical care in general practice, we can no longer ignore - if we ever really did - the call from our patients for counsel and therapy in sexual problems. To achieve even modest success in this complex field of individual practice and human interrelationship, we need some basic understanding of the sexual functions and practices in contemporary society.

Sexual medicine, at least in the Western world, has increasingly made its appearance as a formal teaching topic for the undergraduate medical student curriculum. Formerly fragmented information in the fields of psychology, psychiatry, gynaecology, venereal diseases, community medicine, obstetrics and general medicine have been brought together in a framework which encompasses both sexes and all ages. Many doctors now entering family medicine and general practice have at least an outline understanding of sexuality which they will require to expand further in their surgery and health centre work.

Other doctors longer in practice have not had the benefit of formal student teaching on human sexual experience and sexual problems. They may tackle these problems in a pragmatic way but cannot always be certain of the best outcome or indeed of any modification or cure. They do need a written informing source from time to time.

This book is therefore set out to offer the medical student, the tiro doctor and the more experienced doctor, a general and specific insight into the current understanding of sexual medicine. This writer chooses to offer, in addition, the fruits of his own practical findings in diagnosis and therapy alongside the consensus and practice of a large number of sex therapists whom he respects and admires.

WHAT IS SEXUALITY?

The definition of human sexuality is almost as difficult as the definition of old age. We recognize its continued presence, we know sooner or later how it affects us, we observe many of its external signs and symptoms, we may like or dislike some of what we see, and we know it is a universal feature of mankind. Yet the parameters of its quality and quantity in a given man or woman, at a given time and place, are remarkably variable.

The consensus of folk wisdom - common sense in lay parlance - considers sexuality a natural human instinct, which is frequently channelled into partnership, male with female, and which may encourage conception and procreation, so continuing the generations. Since it is instinctive, sexuality consciously and subconsciously permeates the fabric of our daily lives - in speech, in print, in clothes, in entertainment, in memory, in social relationships, in goals for individuals, for example. Formal religions have long recognized the significance of human sexuality and have invariably found it a suitable place in the ethics, rituals, dogma and acceptable elements of religious practice. In so doing, religion nevertheless makes prodigious efforts to control the instinctive urge and pleasurable gratification of sexuality, by interpretative action.

The secular view of human sexuality takes a less restrictive approach, so that the sexual act can be a source of mutual pleasure and happiness, a psycho-physical expression of mutual need and caring. This can take place within a marital partnership or in a less formal pairing. The link between sex and the possibility of conception is thereby impaired or broken, a result which may have become inevitable with the advent of efficient contraception in any case.

There are a number of received ideas on sexuality in contemporary society, which are *not* in accord with scientific and professional observations, although many lay citizens do continue to hold such notions. They include the following:

Sexuality is only for the able-bodied and those of fit mind.

Sexuality declines rapidly with age, being of little consequence in middle age and virtually absent in senior years.

Sexuality is always within or just below the surface of conscious thought in male citizens but is more subconscious in female citizens.

We are all experts in sexuality once we have begun to experience the drive and outlet ourselves - instinct will always guide us well.

There is a right way and a wrong way to perform sexually (whatever the status of sexual practices in the legal system of society).

Ill health invariably discourages sexuality and, as a corollary, sexual activity can cause relapse or regression of a previous sickness.

Sexual dysfunction implies faulty hormones, body chemicals, or organic defects which a medical doctor can correct with a suitable prescription.

Even if the problem of sexuality is seen to be linked with emotional or psychological disturbance, there is usually some aphrodisiac to correct it.

Sexual deviations - including male and female homosexuality - are not normal or else are actual disease processes.

Hypersexuality in the male citizen is not unusual but in the female citizen (nymphomania) it is rare.

These incorrect ongoing lay views, held singly or in any combination, need to be kept in mind by all counsellors practising in the field of sexual medicine. An awareness of their likely presence will help us both in diagnosis and in therapy of personal and partnered problems.

From the medical angle, human sexuality is envisaged in a physical sense within male or female gender compartments. Both contain elements of an inherited form and elements of an acquired form. Sex is a matter of nature and nurture like so many other aspects of human drive and behaviour. The biological functioning of the man or woman, derived genetically from the sex chromosomes, ensures that most XX inheritors will present suitably female gonads, and XY inheritors will present with appropriate male gonads. With the respective production of oestrogens and progestogens, and testosterone, after puberty, the sex chromosome basis leads to external bodily changes.

The XX holder has mammary enlargement, skin bloom, pubic and axillary hair, ovulation and eventual menstruation and develops the capacity to become pregnant. The XY holder develops penis and testicles enlargement, deeper voice, pubic and axillary hair, general body growth, sperm production and the capacity to impregnate. Of course, genetic anomalies do occur which can modify expectations. (There are two classic examples. XO holders have underdeveloped ovaries and may not become pregnant yet retain a female psychosexual identity. XXY holders have small testicles and penis and a reduced sexual drive. These are the uncommon conditions of Turner's syndrome and Klinefelter's disease respectively.)

By a contemporary paradox, the publicity given to transsexuals ('I am a woman trapped in a man's body') has helped us to review the acquired element in sexuality. The personal view of each of us that we are male or female - an inner feeling of sexual identification - appears to be rooted in early postnatal years. It is subsequently affirmed and reinforced by the attitude and behaviour of immediate members of our family, our relatives, friends and teachers, for example.

THE SIGNIFICANCE OF THE MALE SEX HORMONE

Doctors and midwives in attendance at human birth are accustomed to viewing the neonate and quickly labelling its gender. This depends invariably on scrutiny of the external genitalia. The assigned male or female gender is correct more often than not. Even if subsequent attendance and examination at the postnatal clinic casts doubt on the 'boy' or 'girl' label, no great harm has been done in most cases, except perhaps in the possible problems of birth certification. Of course chromosomal identification for gender would be the ideal but is clearly impractical, in a general procedural sense, for every newborn child.

Experimental work does suggest the possible appearance of gender, and subsequently sexual, intrapersonal conflict, because of the organizing influence of male sex hormone, whatever the *genetic* sex of the foetus. At a high level, presence of testosterone will result in male gender patterns of behaviour - and a lower level will result in a female gender pattern of behaviour.

Testosterone influences or not, we note that gender and therefore sexual behaviour is determined by learned responses. The adventurous and mischievous boy and the homely and doll-loving girl will invariably receive favourable parental and other adult responses to their male and female stereotype, and these are positive reinforcers. Brothers or sisters will be emulated in their recognized male and female roles, further establishing the gender pattern response. In the school setting, segregation by gender will still further reinforce the sense of being inwardly and outwardly male or female. By the sixth year of life -

infant school days - organic and abstract notions of sexual identity are usually complete.

CONTRIBUTORS TO SEXUAL DRIVE

Once we know who we are, sexually speaking, then the arrival of puberty encourages the beginnings of our expression of that awareness. What cannot be forecast in either sex is the intensity of sexual feeling - the sexual drive and need for outlet parallels the spectrum of more 'physical' human parameters; low libido, moderate libido, high libido are acknowledged measures yet cannot be strictly assigned like short height, average height, tall. Testosterone levels apart, we recognize the following factors which may influence basic sexual drive at a given point in each individual's life.

Age of the individual

Kinsey's studies of the American male and female at the end of the 1940s reported maximum sexual drive and outlet in the teens and 20s in men and in the late 20s and the 30s in women. Forty years and many social changes on, there is still considerable truth in these observations. What is significant in terms of the large increase of citizens at the senior end of life, is the absence of any evidence of a fixed end point - in age terms - at which libido simply vanishes.

Presence of a willing and able partner

Individuals who are single, separated, divorced, widowed or widowered can still express their libido in personal sexual outlet through masturbation. The presence of a willing and able partner - marital, casual or paid as the case may be - encourages libido more positively than masturbation, which itself may be incorporated in joint sexual activity. This is well demonstrated in the Newman and Nichols general practice study in North Carolina of the over 60s on their practice lists. Under 10% reported sexual activity in the absence of a partner but nearly 50% were still active when a willing and able partner existed.

Sexual education

This inevitably includes formal teaching or instruction, whether of

5

general biology or human biology or specific lessons at school or college or university; it also includes material learned from media sources such as books, magazines, papers, television, radio and cinema. The sexual knowledge and understanding may be accurate or, especially when learned from peers or even from parents, interwoven with myths, errors and misunderstandings. A clear and specific awareness of personal genital anatomy is too often absent and may become apparent in the sex counselling situation.

Family influence and attitudes

This inevitably links with the previous factor. Discussion on sexual matters may be open and frank, guarded and uneasy, mostly forbidden, or always undertaken with a negative viewpoint. The latter is more often seen in mother-daughter sexual discussions which may arise in the situation of 'warnings to be careful' in first dating events, for example.

Religious influence

In many families and individuals, particularly those with strong ethnic and minority group associations, the religious upbringing, training and attitudes are of basic and ongoing significance. This affects such matters as sex before marriage, conception, frequency, coital positions and the menses, for example. Religious Augustinian teaching is that sex should invariably offer a chance of conception or should otherwise be proscribed.

Preferential sexual experiences

The first ever experience of sexual arousal and the first few sexual encounters are known to influence strongly many subsequent elements of human sexuality in men and women. These include positive elements, like what we find erotically stimulating in vision, smell or touch, and what physical aspects of the opposite or same sex do appeal. Colours, perfumes, music, movements, verbal endearments and street argot which were present at the first stirring of erection or the first sensation of vaginal lubrication, continue to exert a 'turn on' influence in future interpersonal situations. There are also negative influences in that respect, related to first-time sexual experiences. This may include memories of aggression, humiliation, verbal abuse, 'being caught' in a compromising situation, or the discomfort and hurry of a sexual act for fear of discovery or because of cramped situations.

We shall review further elements of influence in basic sexual drive when we come to look at patterns of sexual drive in Chapter 2. In a given man or woman, we may also discover other (less universal) influences that need consideration, for example, interaction with a schoolteacher or youth leader; examples of siblings, gang membership, and being away at boarding school.

THE GP AS COUNSELLOR

In contemporary sexual medicine, there is a wide variety of counselling input. Non-medical sources of aid include:

Newspaper columnists and magazine columnists - the so-called 'agony aunts' and 'uncles'.

Psychologists - clinical, behavioural or educational.

Nurses, and others who are 'trained' in Masters and Johnson techniques

Self-styled therapists - including hypnotherapists, acupuncturists, and others with no obvious formal science training.

Non-medical authors of texts or pamphlets.

Medical sources of aid include:

Family doctors with an obstetrics diploma.

Family doctors with family planning certification.

Family doctors trained by the Institute of Psychosexual Medicine.

GPs with a specific interest in sexual medicine.

Gynaecologists

Psychotherapists with medical degree

Psychiatrists

Specialists in genitourinary medicine (venereologists).

There are ample reasons to view the GP as an ideal counsellor in sexual medicine. These include his having:

7

A full clinical knowledge of his patient.

A full family health and cultural background knowledge of his patient.

A basic trust and confidentiality which the GP's patient can rightly assume in relation to the GP.

An ability to distinguish the organic causes (relatively few in young people but still important) from the psychological causes of sexual problems.

A skill in full clinical and sexual organ examination which I consider is a *sine qua non* in solving sexual problems, whether emotional or physical.

The GP also has the capacity to decide which other medical specialist, if required, is most appropriate for his patient's needs and chances of recovery or improvement. Should such external referral be required, a more effective outcome is likely, since the GP can accept the feedback from the specialist and process the information and recommendations effectively.

Seen from the patient's angle, however, there are also factors which might offer a negative view of the GP as a sexual counsellor. These include:

Embarrassment of the patient where he or she is on a friendship as well as a professional footing with the GP.

Anxiety that the patient's problems may become vaguely or more specifically discussed by other staff in the GP's team and somehow be 'leaked'.

A desire to remain anonymous when seeking help initially instead of being a 'known' patient on the list.

Awareness of the GP's known moral views (secular, religious as the case may be) on premarital intercourse, abortion or sexual deviation, for example.

Fear - in the case of an adolescent or young person - that the information given may be somehow passed on to the parents.

Seeing the GP's age, rather than his professional skill, as a possible barrier to understanding the problem - this can be a young person looking at a senior GP, or a middle-aged or senior citizen looking at a young GP.

A mistaken belief that sexual problems are 'not real medicine for a GP to consider' but should somehow be solved through other help: hence the letters to the 'agony aunts and uncles'.

Any family doctor in practice for a year or more soon becomes aware that, the foregoing objections to him as a sexual counsellor notwithstanding, he will be faced with patients of either sex who have sexual problems that need attention. What is the frequency of such problems in an average practice? There are no useful absolute statistics, for - unlike some illnesses - we are rarely dealing with either a fixed situation or an 'all or nothing event. A European study of a basically middle-class town practice looked at young and middle years adults. One in four men and nearly three out of five women reported problems which included disturbed sexual drive, poor sexual enjoyment, and even total sexual aversion. A Scottish survey suggested that, at family planning clinics, one in five women report a range of sexual problems. In a north-west private psychosexual practice, male first-attenders with sexual difficulties outnumbered female first-attenders by 3 to 1. Non-heterosexual problems may be separated from the general figures so that, at one English psychosexual clinic, one in ten men and one in 50 women presented with homosexual problems.

In counselling, most family doctors soon discover there are recurring patterns in the presentation of sexual upset. We may keep these in mind as we look further at the theoretical aspects of sexuality. They are:

A complaint of poor quality of sexual experience - personal or partnered.

Reduced sexual drive - recent or long-term.

Absent sexual drive - primary or secondary.

Physiological difficulties in sexual response and control.

2
Expressing our Sexuality - and Patterns of Sexual Drive

COMMON FORMS OF SEXUAL EXPRESSION

We are not here talking about merely verbal forms of sexual expression, legitimate or vernacular or argot terms which individuals use to describe sexual acts or use during sexual activity. Words and phrases about sex do, however, crop up in the physical outlet of sexual drive now being considered. Patients explaining and reporting their regualr patterns of physical outlet often do so in vernacular form, rather than in more formal expression. (Caution is required when listening to such local language - terms may be misused, mispronounced or misunderstood by the patient himself or herself. The medical sex counsellor should be familiar with some if not most of these terms, however initially unpleasant they may seem. A table of some of the commoner expressions is appended. (Table 2.1.)

Outlet when alone - masturbation

As Doctor Alex Comfort noted in his book *The Anxiety Makers*, the medical profession was as slow as the rest of the educated classes in recognizing the universality of self-release of sexual tension by means of masturbation. Handling the individual's own sex organs in a vigorous manipulation to achieve orgasm is a feature of both sexes in the unpartnered state. This lone masturbation is commonly undertaken in the following situations:

In adolescence or adulthood, until a partner becomes available.

When a regular partner is ill or absent.

11

When the individual is restricted in choice - for example in prison, in an institution or in hospital.

To complete masturbation to orgasm, most individuals indulge in fantasies, either purely mental or utilizing erotic pictures or other objects, which stimulate the sexual process. These fantasies are often fixed and persistent from early years.

Table 2.1 Common examples of sexual street argot, vernacular and euphemisms

Word/phrase	Some alternatives	"Translation"
Coming, shooting	Spending spunking	ejaculation
Blow job, sucking off	plating, Frenching	fellatio
Scrubber, cert	old banger, easy lay	promiscuous woman
Bumming, browning it	moon shoot, stern one	anal sex
Load, wad	juice, cum	sperm or semen
Pussy, miff	scratch, crack, quim	vulvovagina
Gay, radish	bull dyke, lessy	lesbian
Nuts, balls	bollocks, lunch	testicles and scrotum
Hard on, rod	bone up, horny, full lead in pencil	erection
Jugs, knockers	tits, boobs, melons	woman's breasts

Masturbation is undertaken as a sexual outlet at all levels of intelligence, so that parents or carers of mentally handicapped citizens are often surprised at this performance in those supposedly with no sexual drive or interest. A similar surprise or upset is seen among nurses or carers of older citizens suffering from organic dementia, who expose and play with their sexual organs. This last, however, is an example of disinhibition rather than any positive oriented sexual drive.

Outlet when partnered - masturbation

The presence of an able and willing partner does not invariably imply that sexual activity will be focused on coitus alone. Either partner may enjoy the view of the other in selfmanipulation, approaching or up to orgasmic response. Partners may indulge in mutual masturbation of each other's genitals to orgasm. Such mutual masturbation may take place :

When the couple are unmarried and fear the pregnancy risks of coitus.

When the couple are of the same sex.

When the couple decide on this as a foreplay phenomenon.

When one or other partner is ill or physically handicapped and full coitus is precluded.

When the social circumstances are unfavourable for full coitus - lack of full privacy, absence of comfortable bed, hurried liasons, for example.

While it might be thought that the mere presence of a desirable sexual partner would be enough to arouse and maintain sexual drive during mutual masturbation, for many individuals, an element of fantasing continues to have a significant role. Awareness of this element can be valuable in sexual problems, as we shall see.

Outlet when partnered - coitus

One or both partners (heterosexual arrangement) may decide on sexual intercourse as the ultimate expression of sexual drive in arousal states. A full description of the physiology of the activity phases, which reach a conclusion in intromission of the vagina by the penis, is considered in a later chapter. The prime moving partner may begin with a variety of patterns of sexual foreplay - with caressing of erotic zones, with kissing the lips, with kissing other body parts, for example. This permits fuller arousal of both partners. The partners, for reasons of speed or lack of technique or disinterest in foreplay, may move more rapidly to direct organ within organ placement and begin the stroke play of coitus.

In a homosexual arrangement, female homosexuals may use genital to genital contact with or without a dildo or pseudo-penis or orogenital contact in lieu of intromission intercourse. Male homosexuals may use buttocks masturbation, anal intercourse or orogenital contact in lieu of intromission intercourse.

Outlet when partnered - no masturbation or coitus

Human contact without intromission or genital fondling to orgasm may still provide individuals in a sexual liason some degree of sexual outlet and 'relief' from sexual drive. This is important in many sufferers from physical illness or physical handicap, for example. There are two elements of contact :

Verbal - words of love, expression or praise and endearment, mutual exchange of pleasantries, loving tones in speech.

Physical fondling, caressing, touching, holding.

Once more, either or both partners may use fantasy to achieve more effective enjoyment and relief of sexual tension. This may include, as Baroness Masham has described, the 'memory of orgasm' from the pre-illness or pre-handicapped days - in other words, utilising a psychological orgasm as substitute for a physical orgasm.

Outlet when partnered - alternative or deviational acts

This group of sexual outlets may be incorporated into a regualr sexual relationship for a variety of reasons - stimulus or curiosity, for example. They may also be considered unlawful or proscribed in some partnerships, countries or States. Where a partner is forced to take part in such acts - married or unmarried - the procedure may be classed as criminal and the law will take its course.

Fellation or fellatio is orogenital sex by the female mouth or tongue on the penis and scrotum.

Cunnilingus or cunnilinctus is orogenital sex by the male mouth or tongue on the vulvovaginal area.

Anal intercourse is intromission of the penis into the rectum of the female or male partner or use of finger or fist in the same orifice. This is also known as buggery.

Sadism is use and giving of pain and force to achieve arousal and orgasm - a wide range of apparatus may be used : rope, whip, chain or blades, for example.

Masochism is the receiving of pain and force to achieve arousal and orgasm. Both sadism and masochism may be linked with the use of bondage (tying up, chaining, manacling, handcuffing) and dressing up in special clothing.

Paedophilia or pederasty is the incorporation of a child or under-age citizen in any type of sexual act. This is invariably unlawful.

OTHER FORMS OF SEXUAL EXPRESSION

Incest

Both in a religious context and legal contect, there are severe proscriptions in relation to sexual contact and coitus within a family (other than husband and wife, of course) and among close blood relatives. For many years the incidence of incest was thought to be very low, occurring only among low intelligence individuals or in isolated families or in poor social circumstances. In the last few years, more open discussion of this illegal form of sexual expression has revealed a greater incidence of incest, most often apparently by males - fathers, grandfathers or uncles - and the child - daughter, granddaughter or niece. This may take place unbeknown to the mother or regular sexual partner or, in more extreme examples, with the connivance of the mother to 'keep the peace' with the male partner.

Exhibitionism

This includes a variety of non-contact forms of sexual outlet. Indecent exposure, commonly called 'flashing', usually implies the male citizen purposely exposing his genitalia to passing female citizens of any age. The anticipated response - surprise, horror, 'delight' - arouses the flasher and may permit orgasm.

Wearing clothes which highlight or expose breast or genital zones - male or female - may in a modified form of exhibition be simply part of fashion. In a sexual setting, it may help to arouse and stimulate the male partner who observes this - to erection and even to ejaculation - witness girlie magazine photographs, blue films or videos.

Obscene telephone calls

This is a modern form of sexual expression designed for the caller to achieve arousal and orgasm at a 'safe distance'. The call is intended to shock or sexually frighten or upset the listener thus 'turning on' the caller. There appear to be four categories of caller (usually male caller to female recipient)

The shy, inadequate or immature personality

The psychopathic, maladjusted or antisocial individual

The schizoid, paranoid or obsessional character

The prankster or 'dared' individual, often a teenager or young adult.

The obscene phone caller is also sometimes a depressive citizen for whom this type of call is an aberration from his healthy emotional state.

Such calls are outside the law in the usual way, although it is known that some regular couples, separated for one reason or another, may indulge in mutual telephone endearments of a risque variety. (Some useful approaches in dealing with the nuisance and menace of an obscene phone caller are noted in Table 2.2.)

Table 2.2 Useful approaches to the obscene phone caller

(1)	Keep calm despite the utterance of verbal aggression - a neutral response diminishes the sexual effect on the caller.
(2)	A re-iteration of phrases which negative the call are worthwhile :
	I feel sorry you are ill.
	You genuinely need urgent medical help.
	Does the medicine make you so disturbed?
	Would you like a doctor's phone number now?
(3)	A ironical tone of 'putting him down' is adopted by some:
	Have you thought about a transplant?
	This does not help Brewer's droop.
	That little thing will stay shrivelled.
(4)	Whether arrangements have been made to monitor the caller or not, state:
	Please speak slowly as you are being recorded by the police.
	Can you repeat that for the police tape monitor?
	What is your number, caller?
	If the calls continue, are intolerable and physically threatening:
(5)	Ask the Telephone Service to intercept calls.
	Change your telephone number if possible.
	Go 'ex-directory' even if that seems inconvenient.
(6)	Blowing a whistle, or shaking a rattle, or blasting the caller's ear in any way, is not a helpful deterrent as a general rule; however it may vent the call receiver's feelings.
(7)	In the United Kingdom, British Telecom advises their phone users (in a leaflet 'Nuisance Callers") to put the phone down 'gently, showing no emotion' and avoid long conversations or a trade of insults. 'Most random callers are put off if they do not get the desired reaction.'

Prostitution

The use of a paid partner to release sexual tension and as a means of sexual expression is as old as time itself. (Hence the euphemism 'the oldest profession' for prostitution.) The legality of paid sex - most often female citizen paid by male citizen but sometimes in reverse - varies from one country to another, as do the regulations which cover the illegal format. In contemporary Western societies with a more liberal attitude to sexuality among younger age groups, the business of prostitution has slightly altered in pattern. It still serves visitors and transients in major ports and resorts. More significantly it offers the various deviant forms of sexuality which a regular or marital partner may not offer. It also acts as an outlet for the older unmarried, separated, divorced and widowered (or widowed).

PATTERNS OF SEXUAL DRIVE

We have already considered a number of contributory elements in the sexual drive of humans. These have included male sex hormone levels, chronological age, partner availability and sex education. They also enveloped the influence of family and family background, religious training and beliefs, and preferential sexual experiences. Neither did we discount the possible influences of significant non-parental figures in development such as schoolteachers, youth group leaders, gang leaders and older siblings. Environmental elements cannot be denied either - attending a mixed school or a unisex school, attending a boarding school, 'going away' to summer camps, and even travel abroad with the family, all offer external vistas of behaviours and rituals that may have long-term effects on later patterns in sexuality.

The influence of biological maturity can be seen in age terms. The onset of puberty and progress to adolescence is an era overly filled with exploratory forays into sexual expression, sexual relationships and sexual self-understanding. The degree of intensity in sexual drive - boys and girls - cannot be predicted merely by the degree of beard and moustache thickness or the bust size reached, despite some lay ideas to the contrary. Each teenager can eventually be placed in a temporary category, of minor or moderate intense sexual drive, but this is dynamically affected by other elements: swings of mood, family conflicts, school demands, cosmetic upsets like acne, for example.

Since we live in a youth-oriented society, particularly in Western cultures, and since commerce and industry (especially through advertising) use sexuality and sex drive to sell products, the adolescent finds it hard to escape his or her own sexuality, even if they wished to do so. Music, films, clothes, for example, emphasize sex drive as a positive and significant life element for the young.

In earlier decades, many restrictions precluded sexual drive being patterned in coital forms, and masturbation was more often the norm. Liberalisation of adolescent behaviour and greater freedom of mobility and experimentation have seen a greatly increased coital output of sexual drive in teenage years. This is reflected perhaps sadly in the statistics for gonorrhoea and non-specific disease in this age group and also the incidence of unmarried motherhood. To some extent it has also

17

accounted for greater risk of divorce in the married teenage scene.

Another change has arisen in patterns of sexual drive which may be more apparent than real. In Western societies which once frowned upon (legally and morally) homosexual activity in adolescence and young adulthood, there is greater tolerance of that pattern (morally but not always in legal terms, even between consenting adults). This refers to both homosexual men and homosexual women - the gay community as it is often described. In percentage terms, that pattern may be small, relative to heterosexual patterns but it is often noticeable and vociferous in a variety of ways - through the media and via the political scene, for example.

CHANGED EXPECTATIONS

Among women, the last three decades are alleged to have seen the pattern of sexual drive - in intensity, in variation and in expressed needs - much changed by greater individual and social expectations in sexual partnerships. The women's liberation movement, the women's literary media, the family planning clinics, and the health education programmes have offered information, guidance, encouragement and a positive viewpoint for active female sexuality, with mutual pleasure replacing a passive role with one-sided pleasure.

At the distal end of life, we can again see a changing pattern in both expectations for sexuality and sexual awareness. One example is in relation to the advent of the menopause and the post-menopausal state, Hallstrom's study in the early 1970s suggested that, in the majority of women, sexual interest and orgasmic potential declined following the menopause. This decline was more noticeable in women of lower socio-economic status. To blame this on the hormonal change at the menopause - a variable decline in circulating oestradiol - is not in keeping with the view that male steroid hormone is the key to libido in both sexes, especially since the stromal cells of the ovary, as well as the adrenals, can still produce androgens after the menopause.

Perhaps the suggested fall in sexual interest and orgasmic response is due to problems of a physical sort in relation to local post-menopausal genital changes - vulvovaginal atrophy and lack of lubrication, with reducing evidence of sexual flushing around the labia, discouraging intromission and encouraging dyspareunia. Correction of these by either local oestrogen therapy or by sequential oral hormone replacement therapy may obviate this genital problem and restore sexual interest. In fact, family doctors are aware of requests for help in this menopausal change, by women who do expect and desire to go on with regular sexual intercourse with their partners.

In even more senior years, happily partnered older citizens are no longer prepared to be seen as sexual citizens somehow neutered by arrival at a particular chronological age. The assumption that loss of erectile potency is inevitable past 50 or 60 years is no longer acceptable in an otherwise healthy man with a willing and able wife or companion. As we shall see, this view has extended for some - men and women - even to those, whose illness or operations had traditionally been thought to bring sexual life to a close.

EFFECTS OF ILLNESS AND DRUGS

The effect of illness on patterns of sexual drive is generally believed to be a negative one, especially in the case of illness which is pain-provoking or which produces weakness, fatigue and overall debility. In that respect, absence of drive or reduced drive is often seen by the patient as one more symptom of his impaired wellbeing. Yet this view, oddly enough, may not be communicated to his doctor whose questions are more likely in any case to be directed at other body system functions - lungs, heart or gut, for example. Should the illness recover but the sexual disinterest or faulty capacity linger, then the sufferer may broach the subject to his GP.

The sexual partner on the other hand - who is not ill but who is the carer - may also exhibit loss of drive or interest in sexuality. Here it is either empathy for the suffering of the loved partner or anxiety now acting as a libido suppressor. That anxiety may be appropriate in relation to the information offered by the medical attenders, or it may be fear that if the partner encourages the sick person to indulge in sexual outlet, a catastrophic decline in health or even death may ensue. This last is seen classically after coronary artery thrombosis, especially where there is residual angina. We shall look at the indirect and direct effects of organic illness on sexual function in later chapters.

The direct effects of drugs - legal and illegal - properly prescribed and improperly taken - will also be considered fully later. We must note at this point that drugs influence sexuality as a fctor possibility over the whole age range, from puberty to pensionerhood. Counselling doctors must always have a full 'drugs being taken' dossier of any patient of any age presenting with a complaint of sexual dysfunction.

VIDEO CULTURE

Just as the newsreel showing of local and international acts of aggression or the exhibiting of violent films on television have been blamed, in varying degrees, for a sharp rise of social violence at all levels of society, so changes of patterns in sexual drive and output are now being linked with another form of television, the video film. Many households now have a video machine for the essentially private or family showing of films. Unlike the cinema with its restricted gradings and ability to exclude under-age audiences, the video film is potentially available to all. The sexual content of video films varies from minor and co-incidental in a good and thoughtful movie story, onward through those with a strong and explicit straight sexual content, to films involving all forms of deviational sex, legal and non-legal, moral and amoral. (Cable television parallels this.)

Various legislative Acts have been, and are being, passed to achieve better control of video material and avoid the chance that wrong or inaccurate or deviational views of sexuality be seen by vulnerable or under-age audiences. This censorship may still be passed in a variety of ways, including self-production of video films by partners or partners and friends, with minimal distribution. It may also be thwarted by carefully doctored artistic or educational material, for example.

The video culture and cable television one way or another have given the ignorant, the uninitiated, the routine user, the experimenter and the unpartnered citizen a candid presentation of material. The consequences are neither clear nor meaningful as yet. Neither has it been shown that self-correction of sexual dysfunction has been readily achieved by watching sex videos.

ENVIRONMENT AND OBESITY

Since sexual tension and sexual drive are a dynamic not a static expression of the individual in his daily life, the pattern can be affected by socioenvironmental changes, as well as those elements already considered. This is relevant both to the person who is not in a regular relationship, sexually speaking, and to the man or woman who is married or has a regular sexual partner. This list of influences includes:

Move to a new house/apartment,

Move to a new town/country,

Moving to a housing estate,

Increase in travelling in one's occupation,

Improvement in status and responsibilities at work,

Mixing with a new social set,

Closer contact with attractive staff members, secretary, customers,

Improved personal economic and material situation,

Starting a new career,

Involvement in other sexual arrangements, such as 'swopping',

Regular or heavier gambling,

Drug taking and experimentation.

These influences are functional for both sexes although traditionally said to be greater for the male sex. They also cross all social classes, skilled, professional, manual and semi-skilled, for example, and are indeed cross-cultural and not peculiar to the United Kingdom or the United States.

A final element in this discussion of influences on patterns of drive is the condition best described as obesity. I define this as more than 15% over ideal weight for height and age, or a Body Mass Index greater than 25 (derived from the formula, weight in kilograms divided by height in metres squared). Obesity may be relevant, in six influencing factors:

(1) A cosmetic turn-off (or sometimes a turn-on) to the sexual partner.

(2) Interfering mechanically with sexual positions and sexual stamina.

(3) Encouraging abdominal and pelvic `sagging' with vulvovaginal laxity.

(4) Association with maturity - onset of diabetes and therefore diabetic sexual dysfunctions.

(5) Anxiety and depression, if obseity is undesired and dieting found to be too difficult.

(6) There is a sixth somewhat more positive factor. Mildly overweight ladies in their seventh decade show higher levels of oestrogen than their thinner contemporaries - this lowers the presence of atrophic vulvovaginal changes and loss of lubricatory capacity at orgasm.

Obesity is also associated with organic health problems like chronic obstructive airways disease, hypertension and coronary artery disease. Hygiene is also more difficult for the obese man or woman, not the least in the pelvic and perigenital areas and in the submammary folds. Since these are relevant erogenous zones in sexual play, we can picture the negative influence that obesity may have in sexual relationships. Of course, obesity does not come on overnight and in a stable, warm and understanding relationship, the cosmetic aspect may not affect the pattern of drive very much at all.

3
Coitus in View Today

CURRENT VIEW OF COITUS

Heterosexual intercourse still dominates human sexuality in most societies. All doctors learn the details of male and female anatomy in relation to the reproductive system in their undergraduate course. They usually learn the hormonal and neurological influences which act on the penis, testes, seminal vesicles and vas deferens/urethral pathway as well as those which act on the vulva, vagina, uterus, Fallopian tubes and ovaries. In medical schools with an effective sexual medicine teaching in the curriculum, the tiro doctor will be taught about erectile tissue and erection in both sexes, and ejaculation and orgasm in the man and woman.

Whatever information and additions or corrections that have ensued since their publication of *Human Sexual Response* in 1966, we all continue to acknowledge our debt to the authors of that study, William Masters and Virginia Johnson. Their physiological laboratory studies in St. Louis gave us a firm foundation on which to base an understanding of the complex yet organized processes, which begin with a rise in sexual tension (arousal) and culminate in intromission of the vagina by the penis, with a climax in emission and orgasm. These American studies noted how all body systems - not just the genito-urinary tract - are influenced or involved in the coital act. This is significant in the therapy of sexual dysfunction which we shall consider later.

The four phases of coital activity suggested by Masters and Johnson's research have stood the test of time even if some sex physiologists have telescoped the view into a three-phase procedure. The development is: arousal or excitement phase, plateau phase, phase of orgasm/ejaculation, resolution or refractory phase.

Efferent and afferent flow takes place via the following:

Cerebral cortex, limbic centre, hypothalamus, anterior pituitary.

Autonomic systems - sympathetic and parasympathetic, spinal reflex arc.

Hormone and neurotransmitter systems - catecholamines, testicular and adrenal and thyroid and pituitary hormones.

Other body systems - cardiovascular, respiratory, skeletal, muscular.

Psyche.

The foregoing are incorporated within the coital phases.

Arousal or excitement phase

While awake, this phase may be initiated by actual stimuli from the special senses which are erotically conditioned - sights, odours, sounds, for example, as well as local friction occurring at the glans penis or vulva or simply by body contact and touch. Symbolic stimuli also can produce this erotic effect. The frontal cortex sends initiator messages to the limbic centres (a complex of nuclei encircling the brainstem) and on to the hypothalamus. This is hormonally linked to the gonads and adrenals and thyroid gland. While asleep, dreams can also produce arousal.

Testosterone levels rise, and co-incidentally message ouflows proceed to autonomic outflows. The key noticeable effect is vasodilation of erectile tissue, with engorgement of the penis, of the clitoris and of the nipples at the breasts. A skin flush appears and the labia also flush, as the temperature of the body starts to rise.

An increase in muscle tone in the skeletal muscles is apparent and particularly so in the mammary areas. The TPR (temperature, pulse rate and respiratory rate) begin to rise, and so does the blood pressure in keeping with the catecholamine surge. Gastrointestinal activity is supressed and sphincter action is equivocated.

In relation to penile erection, the main nervi erigentes have been established as the parasympathetic pelvic splanchnics (S2,3, more rarely 4).

Vasocongestion also takes place within the vaginal walls. This prompts the appearance of a vaginal exudate, a lubricatory preparation in addition to the Bartholin's gland secretion which appears in the next phase. Uterus and cervixz are pulled dorsally with a kind of 'tenting' of the pericervical vaginal walls. There is a receptive balloon effect of the inner two thirds of the vaginal wall. Below, some degree of labial parting takes place.

Plateau phase

In this second phase which moves on directly from the arousal phase, there are again external and internal changes. The vasodilatory skin flush of both sexes is now well evident, and the glans penis deepens in colour. The spermatic cords shorten, elevating the testes into the scrotum. Respiration and pulse increase further. Skeletal and involuntary muscle tension also increase, and the rectal sphincter noticeably tightens. Areolar and nipple swelling are more evident.

In the male partner, Cowper's glands secrete into the urethra, and secretion emerges from the male urethra in droplets before any real ejaculation. In the female partner, Bartholin's gland secretion is apparent.

As the uterus elevates with the noted vaginal ballooning, the outer third of the vagina becomes engorged to create an 'orgasmic platform' in anticipation of penile reception. The clitoris is elevated and the labis become more engorged.

The whole picture is that of general and genital preparation for the most significant and sexually releasing phase, ejaculation in the man and orgasm in the woman.

Phase of orgasm/ejaculation

This is the point of coitus in which maximum subjective pleasure accompanies maximal genital activity. Female orgasm involves rhythmic contractions of the outer third of the vaginal barrel and the associated engorged tissue, that is, contractions of the 'orgasmic platform'. The uterus also contracts in rhythmic fashion, and the more intense the orgasm, the more marked the uterine contractions. (These findings have been confirmed by British research physiologist, Dr Cyril Fox, more than a dozen years after Masters and Johnson's reports.) The skeletal muscles also come into play with abdominal, limb, pelvic and even facial muscles in vigorous tension.

Male orgasm is centred in the sensation of being unable to hold the erection without rhythmic expulsion of the semen through the urethra. The semen flows forward as the seminal vesicles, prostate and penile muscles contract in turn. The penis and its urethral bulb literally shoot the semen in projectile fashion into the recipient vagina. The moments before the propulsion are literally described as the 'point of no return' for the male partner. As with the woman, skeletal muscles are fully tightened.

Accompanying the female orgasm and male ejaculation, the blood pressure rises to a maximum and then, just after the climax, drops sharply to a point just below the resting level. Respiratory rate also reaches a maximum of hyperventilation. (Dr Fox noted, however, periods of apnoea during female orgasm, which had not apparently been registered in the St. Louis laboratory work.

The sex flush noted earlier becomes distinct and pronounced and is felt as a pleasant part of the total orgasmic sensation. All observers - lay and experimental - have noted a subjective depletion of bodily sensory activity and awareness of the external environment at the time of orgasmic climax.

Resolution or refractory phase

This may also be called the resting phase, following the vigours and climax of orgasm and ejaculation. In some senses, however, the label is a misnomer. This is because a woman, offered or exposed to further sexual arousal actions, can proceed to one or more further orgasms. The male partner, once ejaculation is fully spent, cannot immediately achieve a 'repeat cycle'. Dependent upon age, experience and other exigencies, sexual stimulation will have no effective response genitally speaking for many minutes up to half an hour or more as the case may be. So there is invariably a refractory or resting phase for the male partner.

In the resting phase in the woman after orgasm, nipple erection diminishes and the sex flush of vasocongested skin recedes. Sweat is noticeable over a wide expanse of the body in one woman out of three but does not seem to be linked directly to the degree of muscular effort during orgasm.

In the genital area a reversal process continues. Relaxation of the vagina's orgasmic platform and descent of the cervix conspire to catch the sperm in the deposited semen in 'unprotected' sexual intercourse. The temperature subsides, the pulse rate decreases, the blood pressure descends to its normal state - these being the changes in both sexes.

In the male subject, the engorged penis returns to its flaccid and relaxed state but in many men its return to the unstimulated 'smaller' size is delayed. (This has sometimes been described as 'partial priapism', although it is not pathological as in true priapism.) Sweating occurs in 30% or more of male subjects as the sex flush recedes. The testes and scrotum slowly or speedily relax. The general feeling of warmth and relaxation may cause drowsiness and even sleep in some partners - not always endearing them to the partner who remains 'awake and interested'.

PHYSIOLOGICAL VARIATIONS

Like the individual partners who join in sexual intercourse, the whole process of coitus has individual elements which add or subtract from the detailed content of the classical four-phase process described above. Here are some examples:

> Slower or faster speed of arousal (influenced by age, health, for example).

> Degree of sex flush and postcoital sweat.

> Variable erectile capacity of nipples, clitoris and penis.

> Variable lubricatory outflow in vagina.

> Single, multiple or absent orgasm in the female partner.

> Faster or slower reaching of ejaculatory climax in the male partner.

These variations may be single or multiple, and well within the range of normality. The partner or partners may not always find such differences from the expected experience acceptable, and regard these as a dysfunction. That is to say, objective and subjective dysfunction may not always coincide for the complaining partner, or the other partner.

COITAL POSITIONS

Partners who form a single and regular sexual relationship tend to favour a particular position or set of positions for penis-into-vagina coitus. Illustrations, oral and written reports from older and modern societies (and countries) show the large number of variations and potential positions that may be undertaken by a healthy and reasonably agile couple. Such positions in contemporary couples become favoured for the following reasons:

> Ease and comfort,

Ethnic or secular or aesthetic acceptability,

Pregnancy or obesity,

Handicaps - physical, environmental.

For some individuals, the first ever coitus and the position adopted - if it produced satisfaction - will tend to be preferred. Others will prefer a variation or experimental approach if not linked to a regular partner, or as part of a personal sexual technique. Cross-cultural studies suggest that the basic most favoured heterosexual positions are: (see Figures).

Face to face, man above woman (Figure 3.1).

Face to face, woman above man.

Face to face, partners lying on the side.

Rear entry to vagina, male partner facing female back (Figure 3.2).

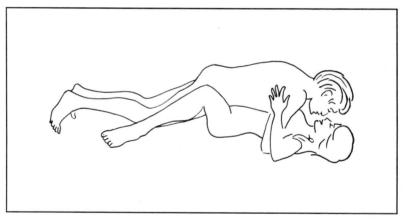

Figure 3.1 Coital position - favourite 'man over woman' in health

A great deal of mythology exists in relation to positions which increase the arousal of the female partner, because of clitoral stimulation for example, or which increase the arousal of the male partner, because of the ability to observe erogenous zones. In fact, all coital positions indirectly stimulate the clitoris, while observational stimulus - or contact area stimulus - varies from one individual to another.

The counselling doctor should be aware of the customary coital positions adopted by the partners, when he is considering reports of erectile dysfunction, or learns of orgasmic difficulties. In illness

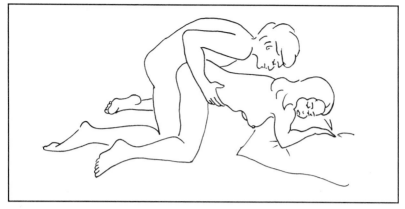

Figure 3.2 Coital position: useful in - poor orgasm (female), obesity, early/mid pregnancy (if acceptable)

associated with disability or with chronic pain, or in pyschological problems associated with cosmetic change, surgical ablation of a part, or in congenital disturbance, the strategies for help may include guidance on coital positioning - how,where, when and with what aids, if appropriate. In suggesting changes from the partners' usual coital approach, the doctor needs to take into account the personalities, education, religious views and rigidity of outlook which may be present. He may need to emphasize that he is giving permission (on health and medical grounds) but that they are not being permissive (in a negative sense).

It has been suggested that coital positioning may reflect not pleasurable experience, not familiarity and not ease of access, but rather reflect the dominance of one sexual partner over another. In the days before women's liberation movements, sexual equality and laws against sexual discrimination, the 'man over woman, face to face,' coital position thereby indicated who was in charge or 'top dog' in the sexual and secular relationship. In today's era of equality and togetherness, we might expect the couple to vary the partner who is on top as a demonstration of this equality. Such a view is difficult to substantiate.

Certainly there are men who insist on being on top, not just in terms of coital positioning but also in being the prime mover for making arousal signals for intention to coitus. Such men may be 'turned off' by a female partner who insists on 'woman over man' coital positioning, or who behaves as the prime mover. Other men do prefer the 'under dog' position and do like the passive role, awaiting first signals from the partner. When encouraged by the partner to be more dominant, this likewise can act as a 'turn off'.

Couples who seek counsel about positioning to improve the chances of desired pregnancy should also be asked about their regular coital positions, in the first instance. Since the uterus and vagina, as we have noted earlier in the four phases description, will change position and shape relative to each other during coitus, the position that offers maximal semen entry, catch and uptake towards the uterus is required. Cervix dipping in a seminal pool is most likely to occur in the 'face to face, man over woman' position, especially if the knees are kept straight as she lies supine.

SOME CONTROVERSIAL POINTS

In the quarter of a century since the appearance of specialist work in the field of sexual medicine - at GP level, in family planning clinics, in psychosexual clinics, in hospital outpatients - the proportion of men seeking help and advice has risen from a handful, to nearing fifty-fifty with that of women. While women have often come alone or sometimes with the male partner, fewer men have come alone for counsel. This changing gender pattern has led to suggesions that:

(1) Doctors who practise sexual medicine should have a co-therapist of the opposite sex. This would permit men to be seen by male doctors and women by women doctors.

(2) Doctors whose counsel is sought by only one of the partnership should always insist that the other partner attends if therapy is to be successful.

(3) When a male GP requires to examine a woman with sexual problems, he should not only have a chaperone present (either, for example, the practice nurse or the woman's partner) but that there should be a woman doctor available in case the patient prefers a same sex physician.

The same view holds for the female GP and the male patient.

Whatever the appeal of these three suggstions, there are no absolutes in the approach to sexual problems. The doctor who is happy and secure in his own sexual identity or in her own feminity, whose personality is fully integrated, whose ability to offer care and trust in a doctor-patient relationship is sound - that doctor need not rely on a same-sex co-therapist for men or women, or insist on treating sexual partners and not one partner alone. An easy and pragmatic style can be just as successful and helpful as any formula-based approach, provided the focus remains the patient's presentation of the problem and the doctor's presentation of being available and willing to ease that problem.

SURROGATES

Another therapy approach along the lines of co-therapist technique, was that considered initially by Masters and Johnson in therapy programmes for some forms of male dysfunction. This was for men who had no available regular partner (single, separated, divorced or whose regular partner felt unable to help sufficiently or effectively. Known as surrogate therapy, the male client was taken under the wing of a girl or woman, who had been trained in the techniques of controlling premature ejaculation, or of encouraging libido, or of overcoming inhibitions, for example.

The woman was not paid directly by the patient but was seen as a member of the therapy staff with a special function and role in rehabilitating the dysfunctional male patient. The ethics of this approach were considered unpalatable by most orthodox doctors in the field of sexual medicine. The woman therapist was seen less as a surrogate and more as a sort of courtesan or call-girl. Many men who entered such therapy welcomed the chance to have an available, trained and - most significantly - fully understanding partner who neither criticized nor blamed them for whatever dysfunction appeared.

Even so, the general feeling eventually settled upon came to discourage the idea of surrogates as possibly adding to the difficulties which partnered, and sometimes unpartnered, men would encounter on returning to their regular sexual scene. This view, plus the ethical difficulties, led to a general abandonment of the surrogate approach except in a few centres of the Western hemishpere. Those who had seen the surrogate therapist as a mere horizontal paid social worker-cum-sensation seeker felt justified in their campaign to stop this approach. Meanwhile the solitary male patient with sexual difficulties, who is given unilateral instruction and guidance, may still seek a paid outlet to 'try out' the counsel.

PHYSIOLOGICAL PUZZLES

The two foregoing points refer to therapy approach in sexual dysfunction. Before we even reach the question of therapy, there are some aspects of the physiology of coitus that remain puzzling if not a little controversial.

We have noted the role of the pelvic parasympathetic nerves in erectile effectiveness. These relate to S2 and S3 and rarely S4, but never all three, in reflex erection. Erection can also be achieved, however, through stimulation of the sympathetic erecile fibres derived from the hypogastric plexus, T10, T11, T12, L1 and L2. This pathway also contains antierectile fibres which require to be inhibited to achieve erection. It is generally assumed that, in coitus, the contact stimulation encourages reflex stimulation of the parasympathetic nervi erigentes whereas, in non-partnered psychogenic arousal, it is the sympathetic hypogastric outflow that achieves erection. The latter mechanism is also at work in the REM (rapid eye movement) sleep phases of the male subject in which arousal and nocturnal erections are known to occur.

When we come to consider erectile failure during coitus, should we assume that in organic aetiology it is the parasympathetic reflex outflow that is invariably at fault, while in the commoner psychogenic block, it is the sympathetic reflex outflow that is inhibited? The difficulty seems to lie in the fact that in any sexual situation, erectile function can be mediated through either pathway. This in turn implies that, in therapy, when we do have sound evidence of an organic source to the erectile fault, we cannot then ignore the psychological management and merely prescribe drugs or ask for a surgical prosthetic implant, for example. The dual mediation of erection in autonomic terms also should make us circumspect, that just because a man still has night erections, is able to masturbate and yet loose erection suddenly, his problem is purely psychogenic.

At the chemical level in terms of neurotransmitters - below brain level - there is still controversy over their influence in the arousal and orgasmic stages of erection and ejaculation. When dopamine agonists were first introduced in the treatment of parkinsonism in the late 1960s, reports of improvement also included reports of recovered libido and erecile capacity in male parkinsonic patients. These were assumed to be a central dopaminergic effect in brain activity. A trial of parenterally administered dopamine receptor stimulants, however, resulted in erection in non-parkinsonic patients. This may imply that the dopaminergic system is involved at central and peripheral levels too.

There are claims in addition that the neuropeptides may have a not fully recognized but significant role in erectile function. For example, blood studies in the contents of the dorsal vein in the erect penis confirm that VIP (vasoactive intestinal polypeptide) appears in high concentration, as it were, in preparation for orgasm. The penile nerves - specifically those of the corpora cavernosa penis - themselves show constant evidence of vasoactive intestinal polypeptide. The identification of other neuropeptides in the vicinity continues, such as somatostin as well as substance P, but not their erectile positive or erectile failure significance.

Possible correction of dysfunction, as we shall see, looks at arterial inflow problems, in relation to the dorsal artery and paired deep arteries, as well as neurological, hormonal and psychological factors. The erect penis also depends on blocking the venous outflow. Here again, neuropeptides could offer an explanantion by way of venous constriction effects and lead us to another erection stimulator approach. Or is venous blockage not achieved by vasoconstriction? Another controversial point that we cannot yet resolve.

4
Common Sexual Problems in the Male Partner

The common things most commonly occur, is a useful aphorism in clinical medicine. It is no less applicable in the field of sexual medicine where experience reveals the recurring nature of some dysfunctions and the relative rarity of others. The latter - like rare syndromes in clinical medicine - often achieve greater publicity than the common and sometimes intractable or difficult forms. For example, most family doctors will have heard of Peyronie's disease but few will ever meet it, whereas dry ejaculation is less familiar yet commoner than the inflammatory disorder of Peyronie.

The traditional and still very useful approach to male partner problems in a heterosexual relationship is to consider a descriptive labelling under one of the following headings.

Erectile dysfunction of primary character

In this state, the young or older man gives a history of failed erection at coitus. Not only may he never have achieved erection for sexual intercourse but he may also never have experienced nocturnal erections, or any spontaneous erections from psychological stimuli, at all.

Erectile dysfunction of secondary character

In this state, the young or older man was previously able to achieve full and satisfactory erection. He now has only partial erectile capacity or else it has become absent for coitus. It may or may not have become absent for nocturnal erections, and for psychological stimuli and masturbation.

Faulty ejaculation

In this state, there are four subheadings - failed ejaculation, delayed ejaculation, premature ejaculation and dry ejaculation.

In failed ejaculation, the man may have achieved partial or full erection for a reasonable time but fails to follow through to the orgasmic stage. In delayed ejaculation, the male partner fails to reach orgasm before or during his lady partner's orgasm and perhaps for some time after, despite a wish to release that orgasmic response. In premature ejaculation, there is nothing dysfunctional about the orgasm itself. It is simply that the orgasm arrives before the point in time which gives coital satisfaction to the man, or to his partner, or indeed to both of them. In dry ejaculation, the man feels to have a full orgasm but no seminal emission is apparent.

Reduced or absent sexual drive and need for output (libido)

In this state, the male partner may have had lifelong poor or absent libido; may have had a healthy libido which has now been affected by physical or mental ill-health; may have been subject to marked fluctuations of libido at different life periods, not obviously related to physical health or environmental disorder.

Drug-induced sexual dysfunction

To these four common and fundamental disorders, we should nowadays add drug-induced dysfunction. This may be either from doctor-prescribed medication, or from taking narcotic or other addictive or self-prescribed psychoactive drugs. Drugs can affect sexuality in all of the four common headings, both adversely and positively.

A number of contemporary studies have sugested alternative practical classifications of erectile dysfunctions. These are now noted in Tables 4.1 and 4.2 and considered in the next chapter.

ERECTILE DYSFUNCTION

A consideration of the common or recurring features of erectile problems throws up, for the physician faced with such problems, a

Table 4.1 Erectile dysfunction classified by 'common factors' (with acknowledgements to Berry and Yorston, 1982.)

(1) Faulty function linked with faulty perennial interpersonal links – the perfect wife or lady on a pedestal
the controlling pseudo-passive partner
the too infrequent or too much in a hurry partner (premature ejaculation)

(2) Faulty function linked with either partner's birth control approach
the blank bullets firer (after vasectomy)
the condom cavalier
the cap or coil IUD lady
the interrupters (coitus interruptus, careful preparers)

(3) Faulty function linked with fear of failure
the once bitten, twice shy
the second marriers
the extramaritals
the easily turned off/poorly turned on
the convalescent
the 'your pleasure matters more than mine' man

(4) Faulty function linked with phobias
fear of being grey haired and past it
fear of self-handling and masturbation effects
fear of operations around the pelvis and genitalia
fear of venereal diseases

(5) Faulty function linked with organic illness
anxiety state, depression, psychosis
genitourinary system disorders
other system disorders

Table 4.2 Ejaculation and orgasm: a time/phase approach

(1) Absent orgasm and ejaculation
 (a) No transport of semen
 (b) Transport of semen but no contractile muscle projection
 (c) Primary form of (a) and (b)
 (d) Secondary form of (a) and (b)

(2) Delayed orgasm and ejaculation
 (a) excessive holding of erection without release ability, which is a lifelong pattern
 (b) as in (a) but intermittent
 (c) Not previously as in (a) but now present and persistent

(3) Inability to delay orgasm and ejaculation
 (a) Pattern from the start of sexual activity
 (b) Intermittent pattern
 (c) Not previously as in (a) but now persistent

(4) Orgasm and ejaculation apparent to man
 (a) Quite satisfactory subjective sensation but no semen appears
 (b) As in (a) but unexpectedly low output of semen
 (c) Poor subjective sensation but some semen dribbles out

a series of partner disturbances which he comes to recognize fairly early on. These upsets of interpersonal relationships, looked at within the context of the long-term history of that interhuman linkage, can be shown to have established themselves early. Once so established, the pattern has continued until one day or one occasion when the man decides to seek help. He may come alone or with the lady partner, to seek counsel.

Faulty interpersonal links

The perfect wife or lady on a pedestal can be a source of erectile upset in two ways:

> She may intimidate her male partner by appearing in a mothering role rather than a lover's role - always there when needed, always supportive and never aggressive, always willing to listen - and, just like his own mother, sexually pure and undefilable.

> She may be rather cold and remote and non-communicative - her clothes, hair, make-up not to be displaced by passion, and her mood to be acknowledged and never over-ridden.

The controlling pseudo-passive partner is a more difficult source of erectile upset. This is the woman who leaves it all, and always, to the man to be the prime mover in sexual activity, and to continue making the running. She may or may not choose to participate fully in the coital process and, when she does, she will have no hesitation in making it clear that he is not matching up to her expectations. This last information by itself would discourage an efficient and potent lover - how much more so a turn-off to the partially erect or failing to erect male partner? Far from being a passive woman, she is an active and aggressive individual, manipulating by negative words and action.

The too infrequent, or too much in a hurry, setting for coitus invites premature ejaculation for the following reasons:

(1) Where the male partner is rationed by his lady partner to only occasional 'agreement' to intercourse (because of her low libido, or organic illness, or her absence at work, for example) then the build-up of his sexual tension may be too great to contain. He therefore reaches an orgasmic peak, and ejaculates, before he or his partner is satisfied.

(2) Where coitus is not taken in relaxed, private situations but clandestinely or in awkward settings, or where intrusion is ever imminent (by children, visitors, parents or regular partners) then

the urgency of the situation is translated into an excess of tension, which explodes orgasmically before he or his partner is satisfied.

Birth control influence

The development of family planning and official clinics in this field revealed a good deal about female partner sexual problems. It also helped to expose the erectile difficulties that may arise in relation to the approach to contraception, unilaterally or bilaterally chosen in the partnership.

Vasectomy invites the male partner to enjoy ejaculation of semen while only - as is said colloquially - 'firing blanks' and not risking pregnancy for his wife. This may promote erectile dysfunction psychologically in three ways:

(1)   Failure to understand the nature of vasectomy may make him fear that he will become impotent - and an emotional block ensues.

(2)   He may subconsciously or consciously decide that now he is 'safe' he can visit other partners, and be turned off by his regular partner.

(3)   His libido may increase as he is 'safe' but his partner rejects this increased interest, so he over-controls.

The condom cavalier is the partner who always has a sheath to hand at the ready but whose erection may fail for four reasons:

(1)   He has to stop during foreplay to don the sheath and this interferes with his build-up.

(2)   His partner welcomes some kind of contraception but invariably claims that the sheath is unaesthetic, uncomfortable or risky, so he is turned off.

(3)   He himself fears that the sheath may rupture and unwanted pregnancy will ensue.

(4)   He has a subconscious venereophobia and wears a sheath as a protection, but is still inhibited by the thoughts of the infection risk intruding on his pleasure.

The lady who uses a cap or some other intrauterine contraceptive device is a well-prepared lady in the birth control sense. This may give both partners peace of mind. It may also for some male partners invite a subconscious picture of the loss of feminity and womanliness which acts as a turn-off. Alternatively, the protected woman may adopt a passive partner role, inviting the male 'to get on with it' and this too becomes a potency inhibitor.

Prior to 'the pill' and safer sheaths, the most popular and cheap approach to birth control was, sometimes still is, the male partner withdrawing from the vagina just before he ejaculates. This coitus interruptus may be encouraged by either partner, or demanded by the lady because it is you that always wants sex so you can take care'. Apart from the risk of pregnancy being high, this interruption just before peak orgasm can lead to inhibition and erectile failure in some men. This will be more likely, when the lady partner places the onus entirely on the male to 'watch it', and thus lower his libidinal pleasure drive.

Fear of failure

In psychologically induced erectile problems, the relevance of fear of failure is all too familiar. The statistic that most men will fail in erection at least once in a lifetime of trying, does little to cheer up those who do so even for the first time. This is especially so where there has never been any thought of failure, and where there is no obvious reason - obvious to the man - why he should suddenly let himself and his lady partner down. This fear of failure may be less marked if a cause does seem obvious - excessive alcohol intake, recent illness, for example. It is also less marked when the lady partner reassures him that there are other ways of pleasure (manual caressing, oral sex, prolonged close contact) and as far as full coitus there is always 'the next time'.

The once bitten, twice shy erectile failure refers to two patterns:

(1)   The man who has never failed before, is proud of his sexual prowess, and is not prepared to chance a repetition of the flop without 'something being done'.

(2)   The man who has failed at even his first efforts in full intercourse, and is quite sure he has a major organic fault which needs investigating.

The second marriage man is doing so after losing his first partner by divorce or by death. He may be marrying a lady who has never married before, or who is a divorcee, or widow. He may fear to let her down in erection because of not having had coitus for some years, or because he might be too excited and ejaculate too quickly, or because he does not match up sexually to her first husband or previous partners. This fear of failure may achieve its effect, and indeed create the psychological block to achieving or holding erection.

The extra-marital relationship may be a one night only experience, a casual and periodic relationship, or a regular liaison. Several factors may induce erectile dysfunction, often unexpectedly:

(1)   A strong sensation of guilt, especially if the pleasure with the extramarital partner is, by comparison, greater.

(2)   A fear of failing to live up to 'unknown' standards of technique or of failure in expectations of pleasuring.

(3)   The partner unknowingly uses turn-off expression, actions or approaches.

(4)   A sudden fear of contracting a venereal illness or of impregnating the woman and making her pregnant.

(5)   Fear that it cannot last, or fear of discovery.

"What turns you off" sex

The easily turned off (or poorly turned on) man may be one and the same individual. The chances of this occurring increase with age so that in middle or senior years, greater stimulus (especially that of contact) is needed for arousal. A man with lifelong low sexual tension levels also fits into this category. Sexual turn-off may result from the following:

Lack of hygiene in the partner

Oral or other body odours

Verbal material uttered before or during coitus

Cosmetic appearance or change -
fat/thin/wrinkled/bald/hairy/sagging/surgical ablation

Lack of female lubrication

Absence of regular stimuli for the man

The poorly turned on man may be lacking in humour, in intelligence, in a sense of manliness, in sexual knowledge, for example, or may have relegated sexuality to an insignificant area of his life goals and daily needs because of career, business, alcoholism, or drug addiction.

Illness and pleasure

Erectile dysfunction in the man convalescing from mental or physical illness may be a new feature of his sexuality, or represent a return to regular problems in this area. Some men, either unhappy with the marital or sexual partner, or themselves of ongoing low interest in sex, may utilize the illness to stop all sexual contact - a sort of laudable excuse for saying no. Some men may have problems over anxiety about straining their 'critical' systems - heart, lungs, blood pressure, for example - because of the effort and muscular exertion of sex. This inhibits erectile capacity.

Some may fear that the illness has robbed them of effective sexual expression, and the fear of failure mechanism comes into play. Others may have failed to receive or ask for expert advice on resuming coitus after a serious illness, like coronary thrombosis.   Careful discussion and reassurance can remedy this.

The 'your pleasure matters more than mine' male partner may see his sexual needs as important, but ensuring the pleasure of his partner in coitus as just as important or more so. Such a thoughtful and caring man may run into the problems noted earlier for 'perfect wife or woman on a pedestal'. He may also spend so much effort, say, in foreplay that his own erection runs out of steam. Alternatively his anxiety to perform well enough to achieve and extend his lady partner's excitement and joy may be an anxiety that creates a mental block after all. This type of pattern can also link with the convalescent male, who wants to keep his lady sexually happy but fears for his health. It may also link with the extramarital partner problems of expectation and technique worries.

Sexual phobias

Irrational fears abound in the whole field of sexuality. They do not need to present with the acute panic states and sense of impending disaster with mass autonomic upset, that characterize say, agoraphobia or claustrophobia.   More often they concentrate on inhibiting the arousal and orgasmic phases of coitus.

The man who is frightened of his changed cosmetic state with age - expressed in awareness of grey hair or baldness, of sagging skin and wrinkles, of less muscular vitality and agility, for example - such a man may consider that he is 'past effective sexual output'. This ongoing myth about age and the notion of a fixed endpoint for sexual desire and sexual output was noted in our opening chapter as one of ten faulty views of sexuality among contemporary lay citizens. It is particularly entrenched as a notion in the under-30 year olds.

Such a view of loss of integrity in sexual terms, in the older man, may be exacerbated if and when his lady partner comments on his appearance or on his performance, or on both. Male sensitivity to partner comments varies at all ages and among different personalities, but the man already suffering erectile dysfunction is hardest hit.

The fear of masturbation, and relieving sexual tension by self or partner handling, may affect erectile function. It has three underlying patterns:

(1) A view that it is 'wrong' to need to masturbate if coitus is practised regularly with his partner.

(2) A view that masturbation reduces the chances of a good erection at promised coitus.

(3) A very ancient view that loss of semen accelerates the ageing process in some indeterminate way so that avoiding erection and sexual output conversely slows the ageing process.

Fear of operations around the pelvis and genitalia may, or may not, be overtly expressed by the man undergoing the surgery. The erectile dysfunction that subsequently emerges postoperatively may be one of four types:

(1) True disturbance of physiological control by operative inter- ference, e.g. after some prostatectomies, after sympathectomy.

(2) Psychological block based on the belief that true disturbance has occurred.

(3) Psychological block based on the fear that coitus will cause relapse (as seen with medical illnesses).

(4) Fear of the lady partner to permit coitus, in case there is relapse or undoing of the operation.

Inadequate knowledge of local anatomy and physiology may add to the irrational fears. The need for postoperative analgesia or other sedative drugs can also depress libido or delay arousal, and such drug effects need to be kept in mind.

Venereophobia has already been mentioned under the condom cavalier heading. Such individuals tend to 'haunt' not only family doctors but special clinics, genitourinary medicine clinics, psychiatrists and even chemists and pharmacists. They may or may not initially have been exposed to the risk of sexually transmitted illness, they may or may not have been treated for that form of illness. An element of depressive illness may accompany venereophobia, and this should be recalled in the counselling and therapy. Both erectile and ejaculatory dysfunctions can ensue from this fear, each psychologically induced. In some men, this fear is part of an obsessional personality problem, so that fear of being less than perfect for the lady partner may also intrude. Definite evidence of venereal illness may not cure the phobia but simply load the anxiety - and erection inhibition - element.

Organic and psychological illness

Anxiety state, depression and psychosis are not physical organic states - as the lower order on Table 4.1 might suggest - but are specific health disturbances which can interfere with libido, erection and ejaculation. Although the lay view is that psychotic individuals, and by analogy all mental patients, are potential 'sex maniacs' or sex deviants, most forms of true psychosis tend to depress the libido in both sexes. Very occasionally, anxious or depressed men do show an apparent increase in sex drive and efforts at sexual output, as if this is an attempt to relieve the anxiety or raise the depressed state by once-much-enjoyed activity.

Loss of sexual interest, and associated erectile difficulties, may oppositely be an early sign of neurosis or depression. This is especially so if there is a sense of guilt about pleasure for 'unworthy' or 'wicked' individuals, a self-assessment that may turn up in the depressed man. Sexually inappropriate behaviour may be seen in schizophrenia, but this need not include evidence of erectile dysfunction. Organic dementia, presenile or later arteriosclerotic, can produce erectile dysfunction whether the libido appears normal, lost or excessive.

Therapy of anxiety and depression, by psychotherapy and appropriate medication, should expectedly see a return of libido and effective erectile function, as these emotional complaints steadily resolve. Unhappily, the drugs used - tranquillisers, thymoleptics - may themselves centrally or peripherally affect the reflex nerve function, interrupt the pathways flow in arousal and orgasm, and produce complaints of loss of potency for erection and/or ejaculation. Such a complaint calls for a reappraisal of both dosages in use, and the possibility of substituting the drugs being given.

We should recall that the erectile failure itself may be the source of either the anxiety or the depressive state. The latter state, depression, is mild to moderate and there are few reports of severe depression, inducing a risk or attempt at suicide, because of sexual dysfunction alone. To the anxiety or depression may be added, after a succession of partial erections or inability to hold erections, a cumulative fear of failure. This in turn exacerbates the problem.

We shall look comprehensively at the significance of systemic organic illness on sexual function later in this chapter. Here we can list the more significant of such illnesses. Effects may be short or long:

Bacterial and non-specific urethritis
Chronic prostatitis
Orchitis - traumatic or infective
Lumbosacral/hips osteoarthritis
Diabetic polyneuropathy/infective or toxic polyneuropathy
Arteriosclerosis - pelvic vessels, coronary or cerebral vessels
Corticospinal disorders, e.g. parkinsonism, demyelination, 'stroke'
Asthma and chronic airways disease
Myocardial disease/coronary artery ischaemia/chronic cardiac failure
Postoperative states
Life-threatening illness
Chronic renal failure
Hormonal deficiency states

The figure of 10% of cases, given as the percentage of organic incidences of sexual dysfunction in men, rises steadily with the years. By the sixties, it may be 15-20 and after 75 years, organic illness tends to dominate the picture, even if it is often mainly degenerative in origin.

EJACULATORY DYSFUNCTION

Absent ejaculation

While discussion continues on the question of whether male orgasm is one complete phase, or is in two parts - a collection and an expulsion (sometimes called emission phase and contractile phase), the disturbance of ejaculation can be better explained by the 'two part' viewpoint. For example, a very old man may experience absence of ejaculate yet be aware of a feeling of orgasm If we assume that arteriosclerosis and/or hormone deficiency has denied ejaculate production, we can explain this phenomenon.   No semen was transported to the prostatic urethra (between the external and internal sphincters) but there was reasonable contraction of the bulbo- and ischiocavernous muscles as well as skeletal muscle contracture of the back and limbs.

A hypertensive young man put on an autonomic inhibitor for control of blood pressure might offer a parallel picture. The drug blocker reduces seminal fluid secretion and movement to a minimum but does not inhibit muscular action. In both the young man and the old man, memory of previous unsuccessful orgasm also adds to the psychological pleasure anticipated in the present but dry coitus.

The transport of seminal fluid to the prostatic urethra may not be followed by pubo- and ischiocavernous muscle contraction. Instead, the column of liquid is passively dribbled towards the penile tip and then seeps out steadily thereafter. A sensation of orgasmic relief may or may not be experienced We may assume to be present either a neuropathy (for example, B vitamin deficiency or alcoholic in aetiology) or else diabetic neuropathy or lower cord lesions. In post urethral dilation in stricture derived from venereal infection or after trauma, for example, this phenomenon may make its undesired appearance. Acute urethritis may occasionally produce a parallel picture, if coitus is attempted.

Delayed ejaculation

Excessive holding of erection without the ability to release the ejaculate and orgasm at the point desired (by the man or his partner) used to be called, indeed may still be described as, retarded ejaculation. This semantic label is almost as sad as the traditional terms impotence and frigidity, applied to men and women, whose very name reeks of permanent failure and irreversible status. Far from being retarded, the man is perfectly rational and his needs are just as positive as the next but he is in the position of faulty timing (sometimes known as overcontrolled) orgasm.

This orgasmic delay may present in the start of his sexual life and stay with him. Alternatively, the delay may appear at a later stage in his sexual progress. A look at the possible triggers to overcontrol or delayed timing reveals the following possibilities:

Need to wait for partner arousal which is much slower than self.
Anxious to hold until partner is ready to orgasm.
Dislike of a particular position, insisted on by the partner or by the environmental circumstances.
A strong sense of guilt at the pleasure being enjoyed.
Cryptic homosexuality in a male/female partnership.
An extension of the 'woman on a pedestal' syndrome seen in erectile dysfunction.
A need to prove his virility in 'holding on'
The use of coitus interruptus as a contraceptive approach
Greater pleasure in masturbation than coitus
Need for the presence of a sound, word, smell, fetish, to 'release' the reflex
Partner dislike if alternative orifice used - mouth, anus, for example, in heterosexual coitus.

In the primary form, the first ever occurrence is likely to establish the pattern, and this is positively reinforced as the years go on.

Premature ejaculation

The most familiar and best-known form of ejaculatory dysfunction is still popularly labelled 'premature ejaculation'. Some sexologists have suggested that this label is incomplete in that it refers only to the expulsion phase of the sexual act and not to the orgasm as a whole (which includes the seminal collection phase organically and the emotional phase psychologically). Some men who complain of premature ejaculation would seem to have begun their sexual life, inexperienced and immature, with a holding back difficulty, which reappears in each new relationship. Some only complain of this problem on an intermittent basis and can relate it to a particular event or activity - for example, after too much alcohol, or when anxious about forthcoming events like exams or an interview or a competition. A third group have rarely or possibly never experienced this but, in a new partner situation, or after a long period of abstinence from coitus, develop it as a persistent and disturbing fault.

The definition of 'premature' is often a personal one - of needs, expectations, desires - or a partner one, along the same lines. To limit the definition to one of time from arousal to ejaculation may invite invidious comparisons and cause unnecessary anxities for the man and his partner. As a working useful yardstick, Bernard Goldstein of San Francisco State University has suggested this definition:

A man who is unable to hold back from ejaculation for at least 60 seconds after the penis enters the vaginal orifice.

The problem here is that some men consider it a 'virile performance' if they have fast arousal, and a quick intromission and ejaculation. This self-styled macho partner is more usually ignoring the needs, wishes and interests of his lady partner when he acts in such a 'dive in, dive out' fashion.

Behavioural approaches have offered much help in this particular form of ejaculation difficulty, as we shall see later on. We have to recognize, however, that this upset may not be invariably psychologically derived and augmented by positive reinforcement. Diabetic neuropathy not only produces erectile dysfunction but can also result in ejaculatory miscontrol, including the premature expulsion of semen before the couple are mutually satisfied. While diabetics can have psychological problems too, there is a need to exclude neuropathy in this category of patient. Such patients are more refractory to therapy than those with erectile disturbance.

By a curious turn of events, the list of trigger mechanisms already outlined as a possible source of delayed ejaculation can be responsible for the appearance and persistence of premature ejaculation. Not only, for example, coitus interruptus and slow arousal in the lady partner but all other elements - guilt, orifice presence, position of coitus, woman on a pedestal and cryptic homosexuality.

It should not be forgotten that 'local' problems may encourage long-term or short-term premature ejaculation - for example, infection of urethra or bladder from bacterial invasion, balanitis, vulvovaginitis. The presence of a scrotal hernia has been blamed. Orchitis can be a factor, whether viral or bacterial. The condition may be seen in convalescence after illness or surgery of an individual and may then be related to fatigue, weakness or anxiety about health generally, or recurrence of the complaint - mimicking the problems in erectile dysfunction.

In some men, the problem is self-correcting, as a new partnership 'settles down', or the couple obtain privacy and relaxed surroundings. There is no guarantee, however, that familiarity will assure a cure.

Reduced ejaculate

Orgasm and ejaculation may be enjoyed subjectively and be apparent to the male partner but the female partner has an absence of seminal flow sensation in some instances. This latter may arise because there is literally no outflow of any 'stored' ejaculate in the prostatic segment of the urethra. Alternatively, there may be a reduced or very small flow of ejaculate.

Reduced ejaculate is noted in four circumstances:

Slightly so, after vasectomy, in some men
Falls between 30 and 60% after the age of 65 years
Chronic prostate inflammation or disease of seminal vesicles
Primary or secondary testosterone deficiency

The ejaculate may also be reduced after a high frequency of coitus in a given 3-day period. To assess reduction, the man should abstain for a 3-day period (up to 6 for older citizens) and then measure the ejaculate. A figure that is below 0.5ml would confirm marked reduction.

Another source of absent ejaculate is the so-called retrograde ejaculation. Here again, the male partner enjoys the feeling of orgasm but no emission takes place. When emptying the urinary bladder later, sperm or seminal material may be evident. This implies that during the expulsion or contractile phase of male orgasm, the internal sphincter functions inappropriately and the ejaculate leaks into the bladder, and not forward propulsively through the urethra into the vagina. Retrograde ejaculation may be a primary malfunction or it may appear at any time in sexual life. The aetiology is often unclear, although it is alleged that diabetics are more at risk to such a sphincter malfunction. It may also take place after prostatectomy operations or cystoscopies, and dilation for stricture. Very occasionally it may be drug induced, and withdrawal of the offending medication reverses the process.

The last category in Table 4.2 considers the man with poor subjective sensation of orgasm although plentiful or some semen dribbles out. This loss of orgasmic pleasure and excitement may be partly psychological, especially if the reduced ejaculate is felt to be a sign of diminished virility, or there is expressed loss of expectation by the lady partner. We have already noted earlier in this section the possible organic sources - with or without emotional aspects, of the dysfunction: acute urethritis, prostatitis, diabetic neuropathy, poststricture dilation and drug-induced forms.

ALTERED LIBIDO

From what we have seen of the acquired nature of sexual drive, levels of sexual tension and need for sexual outlet, we already have concluded that libido is nowhere a fixed aspect of human activity. It is dynamic in positive and negative directions, and can be influenced so by single factors or multiple elements from within and without the human body and mind. We have also suggested a familiar pattern of intensity is present within each man, which can be incrementally depressed or elated but tends to be ongoing as 'high, moderate or low' in a relative fashion. Such labels tend to be useful only for comparison within life phases of a given individual, and are less significant or useful for comparison among several individuals. There is a risk of raising expectations or adversely influencing progress, when we listen to a man's sexual history or problems then openly evaluate whether his sex life is good, moderate or bad. When he finds a partner who reasonably matches his wants and desires, he is more likely to be successful in his sexuality, other matters being equal. So often, counsellors in sexual medicine recognize the presence of libido incompatibility in partners.

ANXIETY EFFECTS

In younger and middle years of life, alteration of libido is more often psychologically derived than organically. Stress and anxiety in any life circumstances - at home, school, college, workplace, for example - can depress libido. The stress may arise from adverse circumstances - money problems, overcrowding, failing exams, lack of employment, difficult interpersonal relations - or paradoxically from successful circumstances - sudden fame, goals all achieved, sudden riches, increased respinsibilities. The anxiety may derive from a wide range of areas:

Health of self, of family, of friends
Expectations of self, of family, of friends
Change of circumstance, as in moves to new job, new town, new country
Alteration of family - getting married, having a child, loss of loved one
Fear of ageing, fear of cosmetic change
Loss of job, retirement, menopause, male climacteric

The lifelong anxious personality appears more sensitive to external events and circumstances increasing depressing effect on libido. Greater distractability, increased sense of fatigue, lower pain threshold, for example, are intrusive elements in any level of sexual drive, and all three are linked especially with the anxious and tense individual.

Organ size

Anxiety, as we have noted earlier, feeds on itself, in relation to erectile and ejaculatory dysfunctions. One episode is enough to trigger anxiety over future failures. This fear of failure in turn can depress libido and create a self-fulfilling prophecy of the event - such anxiety can be augmented by criticism from the partner, or by the sufferer listening to his workmates boast of their alleged virility and constant success in intercourse.

Another anxiety that may lower libido concerns penile size. This is more likely in the sexually inexperienced man although not necessarily so. For example, a woman with laxity of the vagina may receive less pleasure from a smaller organ and may say so. The previously unperturbed and experienced male partner then loses confidence. Instead of persuading his lady partner to seek help - through vulval and perineal exercises or even by way of a 'tightening' operation - he seeks help from his family doctor about his too small organ. Sadly, unless he was suffering from true hypogonadism or perhaps incomplete erectile function, there is no successful way of augmenting the width and length of the flaccid penis. This has not stopped efforts by charlatans and romancers in offering a whole range of approaches and techniques, offering the user or participator a 'really big organ', starting with his basically self-assessed small one.

No one denies that, rarely, a microphallus is observed, or even, in a true hermaphrodite, a small unattached phallus. Most men who suffer true anxiety and even a full-fledged neurosis about the size of the penis, are doing so on the basis of one or more of the following incorrect notions:

The man who achieves most sexual attention, and can give maximum sexual satisfaction, is the man with a large non-erect penis and an enormous (length and girth) erect penis.

The man whose penis is apparently small - seen from above, so to speak, or in a mirror - may be a latent homosexual or may be a male deficient in male hormones.

The man with a small organ can never bring his partner to orgasm.

The man with a small organ may never be able to father a child.

Such notions may be spoken aloud or be held covertly and so produce anxiety. They may be aggravated by direct observation of men while swimming, bathing, in public conveniences or seen in photographs or films. Such men may be unaware that making love in a cold environment or under pressure of 'discovery', for example, can keep the penis in a poorly engorged 'smaller' state.

Libido may be affected by an underlying sensation of guilt which raises its unhappy head in such circumstances as:

Continuing to enjoy a sexual partner when a best friend has lost his.

Continuing to indulge in coitus when a close relative or friend has died.

Continuing to seek out female company soon after a divorce.

Finding a need for outlet soon after a major illness or operation.

Finding sexual attraction in younger women when turned off by a partner of one's own age.

Hypersexuality

Libido can, it should not be overlooked, also increase in its intensity.

This change in an upward direction is given various labels, including hypersexuality (applied to both sexes), nymphomania (women) and satyriasis (men). This condition is often viewed as unlikely to be other than mythical, so common is the opposite state of low or absent libido. Alternatively, hypersexuality may be viewed as merely a relative (not absolute) state when the libido of one member of a partnership is matched with that of the other. While this may be agreed in some individuals, there do seem to be six examples of hypersexuality which can be considered in a more absolute sense:

(1)   Sexual drive linked with violence or criminal action - the individual man is unable to control powerful sexual needs in a social and legally acceptable manner.

(2)   Sexual drive linked with disinhibition which is not psychopathic - this may be the effect of drugs affecting cerebral function, or the effects of presenile or arteriosclerotic dementia.

(3)   Sexual drive in a 'rebound' effect after depressive illness or after a life-threatening illness.

(4)   Sexual drive augmented by a frustrating partner who has low libido, or is anorgasmic yet otherwise loved.

(5)   Sexual drive linked to institutional restrictions - as in prison.

(6)   Sexual drive altered by schizophrenia

There is no real evidence that either male or female prostitutes can be categorized under the hypersexuality label. This had been suggested as one of the reasons why such women (fewer men) follow this path as a way of life and earning a living, that is, to mollify and satisfy constant sexual urges while ostensibly offering a service to the needy or curious.

A fine line can be drawn between promiscuity and hypersexuality in considering libido. For example, a high sexual drive and output contained within a single partnership or perhaps with an alternative partner only, would be reasonably labelled as hypersexuality. The individual man or woman who has multiple partners, random as well as regular, opportunistic as well as arranged, would be reasonably labelled promiscuous. As well as numbers of partners, there is the frequency of sexual acts with each partner so that, in theory, if a man has eight partners but only has coitus once with each, he may be viewed as promiscuous rather than hypersexual.

Promiscuity is significant for the doctor who is trying to control the spread of sexually transmitted diseases. Hypersexual states are significant for the doctor where:

(1)   Counsel is sought by the partner who cannot cope with her hypersexual man.
(2)   Counsel is sought in hypersexuality of dementia or drug dependency.
(3)   Counsel is sought in schizophrenic disorder.
(4)   Counsel is sought in delinquency or other antisocial behaviour.
(5)   Counsel is sought by the hypersexual individual who wants to limit or control his needs.

It is possible for hypersexuality and promiscuity to be combined in one individual and this creates considerable 'management' problems in relation to disease control, for example.

DEVIATIONS AND DIFFICULTIES

Bisexuality

So far we have considered only heterosexual drive, relationships, and possible dysfunctions. We can look shortly at homosexual sexuality in its various formats. Before doing so, we might usefully take up the deviation from total heterosexual state, known as bisexuality. This description should not be confused with that of hermaphroditism. The bisexual citizen (in street argot, once known as AC/DC) has a full male genital apparatus and a naturally male biological profile. He claims, however, that he is sexually oriented toward men and women, and not exclusively and continuously heterosexual or homosexual.

This personal view of oneself as bisexual presumably takes in the three aspects of choice of sex partner:

A leaning or preference to neither sex
An ability to be stimulated emotionally and physically by either sex
A refusal to be categorized as homosexual or heterosexual.

To be able to claim bisexuality, the man must have had same sex experience and contact as well opposite sex intercourse. Unless such experiences and contacts were very evenly balanced over a given period of time, we might suspect that at least some claimants to bisexuality were preferentially heterosexual because they were uneasy, anxious or socially unhappy about homosexual behaviour. This would explain married heterosexuals (presumably fully committed to a one partner (woman) relationship) who undertake intermittent or regular homosexual extramarital relationships.

We might also perceive bisexuality as a 'phase' of shorter or longer duration, when a man is moving from the heterosexual to the homosexual pattern of sex life or, less commonly, vice versa.

Homosexuality

Not withstanding the biological structure of man and woman and the need for procreation in biological terms, and despite the normative teachings of religion, culture and education in a dominantly heterosexual world, homosexuality has appeared in all social groups and civilizations down the centuries. The homosexual man or woman (sometimes described respectively as male invert or lesbian respectively) shows partner preference for the same sex, is emotionally attracted to the same sex, and may in turn undertake physical contact in a sexual format with a member of the same sex. In a country where homosexuals are in the minority of the population, they are viewed as sexually deviant from the heterosexual majority. Those who subscribe to the view that homosexuality is a pathological state in a man or woman, have no hesitiation in classifying homosexual preference and behaviour as 'just one more sexual deviation'. Those who view homosexuality as one of the gradations of sexual relationships in mankind, take a more tolerant stance. It then becomes just another variety of human behaviour in an emotional and sexual context.

Over 40 years ago, the studies of Alfred Kinsey in the United States of America revealed the (then) startling fact: 37% of adult males admitted to one or more homosexual experiences in their sexual life. This was not just individuals who had been 'confined' to all male settings - boarding schools, armed forces, prisons, for example. It did include adolscent sexual experiences, and it did include many who later settled to heterosexual relationships and remained heterosexual. A current estimate of homosexuality in the English scene suggests a figure of one in 20, mostly overt, homosexuals in the society.

The nature of homosexuality - is it genetic and therefore predisposed, or is it acquired, or is it a combination of nature and nurture - has not been agreed either by interested professionals in human behaviour or by practising homosexuals themselves. The attitude of non-homosexuals varies from country to country, from decade to decade, and across the generations. It may be viewed as a normal variant of sexual behaviour, an abnormal variant or deviation, a mental-cum-physical disturbance analagous to a psychosis, a form of moral degeneracy, an antireligious practice, and an antisocial behaviour pattern.

Whatever the possible genetic or intrauterine fetal influences, environmental studies suggest that families with an 'absentee father' show a higher likelihood of homosexuality in the sons. This applies not only where the father is physically absent but also where he is apparently disinterested and emotionally indifferent to the son. Less evidently influential but sometimes quoted as an environmental factor is the overprotective and emotionally intense older mother (older in terms of a woman's reproductive period).

Another suggested environmental influence is the effect of preferential sexual experience, where such experience is that of an encouraged overt homosexual act, or stimulation by observing the naked male body in whatever circumstance. Alternatively, initial heterosexual experience may be so unpleasant or unrewarding that a trial of homosexual experience is undertaken and then repeated. Homosexual preference may be encouraged by mixing in a homosexual clique socially or by entering occupations where homosexuality has long been permitted as acceptable - for example in the entertainment industry, in the hair, beauty and cosmetics industry, and in fashion concerns.

The individual reaction to the personal discovery of preference for and sexual arousal by the same sex, leads to a variety of reactions in a given individual - increasing tolerance of homosexuality (the gay community, in street argot) notwithstanding. One homosexual may try to suppress his feelings and needs, adopt a heterosexual external stance, and remain covert in his wishes despite any personal anxiety or stress ensuing. Another homosexual makes a steady and satisfactory acceptance of his preference and emotional responses, openly revealing his needs and seeking out a partner of similar form of homosexuality, tending towards a 'feminine' format of speech, dress and attitude while also seeking out a like-thinking partner.

The first pattern individual may indeed cloak his homosexuality by taking on a wife as partner, and procreating, to give a family stabilty to his heterosexual façade. The woman may be aware of his homosexuality and join in the social charade while tolerating covert homosexual behaviour. The woman may alternatively be unaware of her husband's true sexuality, and discover it merely by chance or only when the husband can no longer tolerate his own 'hypocrisy', as it were.

Since homosexual intercourse is either by way of oral sex or anal sex, the possible dysfunctions for which a homosexual man seeks guidance still include erectile and ejaculatory dysfunctions much on the patterns already discussed. Physical disorders of the anus - laxity, tears, inflammation, for example - may also bring the homosexual for counsel. Currently the most common reason for attending the GP is the question of exposure to sexually transmitted diseases but most especially to the AIDS virus, HTL VIII.

Female homosexuality

In the United Kingdom, in the late 1960s, the figure given for admitted female homosexuality (lesbian or gay woman) was 1 in 40 of the female population. Earlier American studies suggested that one in seven women had a homosexual experience at least once in their lives though not necessarily settling into a lesbian existence. Contemporary statistics in homosexuality fail to give a clear picture of sheer numbers but the coming of the 'gay liberation' and the women's liberation movements has permitted a more open expression of same-sex feelings in the female community.

As with male homosexuality, many theories are forwarded on the reasons why a particular girl or woman comes to orient herself sexually towards the same sex. Helen Deutsch offered the view that a woman may reject 'men in general' because of vicious or cruel behaviour on the father's part during her childhood. Another view suggests that homosexuality of the lesbian pattern indicates an internal physical failed equilibrium of male and female sex hormones at a critical point in psychological development. There is no objective proof of such an imbalance, even in the so-called butch lesbian who talks in manly fashion and wears paramasculine costume.

The influence of the absentee or hostile father, allegedly of significance in male homosexual development, may have a parallel in lesbian progress. The budding girl is likely to take her mother as the model of her future womanhood. If that mother is warm and loving towards the father and shows fondness for, and pleasure in, her children, then traditional feminine roles are present. Female homosexuality may then derive from a disturbed maternal model, the mother being absent or chronically ill or a negative figure in relation to the father and the growing children. Faulty identification may be present with aunts, teachers and youth leaders as well.

Female homosexuality in its formal expression of love and sexual drive towards the same sex is said to affirm a 'mother–daughter' (woman to woman) relationship which the girl had never experienced when growing up, and each act of love and affection is a subconscious re-enactment of that missing bond.

There has always been a strong contrast between the heterosexual community's attitude to female homosexuality and that towards male homosexuality. The former has long been more tolerated and accepted if for no other reason than the many non-sexual companionate couples of women who make women 'living together' respectable in heterosexual eyes. The view of lesbianism has also been considered less harshly because, so it is thought by heterosexuals, there is no 'corruption of youth' or strong link with pederasty as in the matter of male homosexuality.

Request for counselling in homosexuals

The family doctor may be approached by the homosexual man or woman, or by the parents of young homosexuals, or even by the partner of the homosexual for the following reasons:

A wish to talk out his or her feelings and sexual orientation.

A request for help in 'changing' to an heterosexual.

A desire to enlist the doctor's support in condemning the gay son or daughter, and coercing a therapy to change that sexuality.

A request for drugs or therapy to help with depression, anxiety, or panic - or else to 'suppress' homosexual desires.

A request for the doctor's aid in contacting the homosexual helping groups like CHE (Campaign for Homosexual Equality) or various ethnic gay groups.

Anxiety to determine if he or she may have developed or be carrying the HTLV III (the 'AIDS') virus.

The doctor or any counsellor of young gay people must keep in mind the legal picture while nevertheless offering maximum guidance and support.

There are continuing claims that homosexuality is a pathology that can be 'treated or cured' but scepticism is appropriate at all times. Various therapies that have been applied include full psychoanalysis, short phase psychotherapy with insight orientation and environs adjustment, aversion and desensitisation techniques, and even hypnotic and tranquillizer therapy. The end result rarely, if ever, justifies the means.

Help can never be given to the homosexual by offering 'good advice' like 'it is just a phase' or 'get yourself a boyfriend (or girlfriend)', or even 'try having a baby'! Neither, despite the mentioned theory on hormone imbalance, is there any justification for giving male or female sex hormones. Some homosexuals only just appear in the surgery (the threat of AIDS virus apart) for medication of transmitted diseases, and may not even indicate their sexual preference, though anal infection in a man will give that preference away (homosexual or bisexual).

Sexual aversion

In the United States, sexual aversion has come to be considered as a distinct, if not always distinctive, syndrome in sexual dysfunction. Such aversion can affect both sexes, and is most pointed in direction when the sufferer experiences a powerful antipathy to human contact which might or is likely to proceed towards sexual acts or sexual play. The key element is - like those with a phobic state - to avoid events, situations, verbal interchange or physical proximity which could offer or invite an opening touch taken as a message of intent.

The aversion may actively create a sexual dysfunction in the sufferer or in the partner, or alternatively be a consequence of a sexual fault or difficulty in the sufferer or the partner. Obvious examples include failing erection, premature ejaculation, and experience of painful coitus as a *post hoc* or *propter hoc* stimulus to aversion. On the other hand, sexual aversion may stand alone - and very puzzling or upsetting to the partner - in its presentation as a dysfunction. In such cases, the aversion may mistakenly be labelled as depressed or absent libido, or a feminine 'frigidity', or even as indicating sexual inversion (potential or actual homosexual preference).

The San Diego sexologists, R.T. and T.L. Crenshaw have suggested there are two forms of aversion which can be separated out of the format. In secondary aversion, the freeze on contact is directed towards the current sexual partner, but need not be an aversion to other actual or potential partners. This is more likely to appear in women than men. In primary aversion, commoner in men, the antipathy to contact is set against all partners, actual or potential. It is frequently accompanied by other forms of sexual difficulty, such as erectile dysfunction or anorgasmia.

If aversion is seen as an anticontact phobic state, then we can understand that the degree of phobia may be mild, moderate or severe. We can also understand that a medical counsellor in sexual dysfunction may be faced with a disappointing failure of outcome, when a specific problem is suitably tackled, say, the squeeze technique controls too early ejaculation, but the phobic state of aversion to contact has not also been recognized and tackled.

Accepting that there are, as the Crenshaws designate them, primary and secondary sexual aversive states, we might surmise that the secondary phobia would be readily amenable to therapy but the primary phobia would be less so. This does in fact prove to be the case, as we shall see later. This also implies that the individual presenting with secondary aversion has almost certainly been part of a strong, physically active, emotionally charged interrelationship, mostly likely in a marital context. This itself offers hope for therapy and reconciliation. For the non-marital or poorly bonded couple, the situation is more tentative.

The personality type most likely to develop secondary aversion can be introvert or extrovert overall, but is often either a hypersensitive character, easily dismayed or disturbed by events, or else a mildly depressive individual, who is unsure of his or her own sense of worth and self-significance. Having said that, even brash egotistic characters and loud self-confident individuals may find they begin to react phobically to a partner's touch threatening further sexual advances. This itself may upset their self-confidence and assuredness, and make them begin to question themselves in a wider sense than merely sexual - or lack of sexual - responsiveness.

Transsexualism

This is a psychological problem initially, not to be confused with inter-sex states based on pseudohermaphroditism. Most commonly in XY males who develop feminine feelings ('female trapped in a male body'), the thoughts turn in this direction well before puberty. It is not therefore the result of being turned on, or turned off, by a sexual encounter. Nor is it any alleged effect in which, as adolescents, the young men are subject to homosexual 'seduction'. A look at the behaviour in prepubertal years - hobbies, toys, dressing, play-acting - as seen throught the man's eyes, or his parents' eyes, suggests the presence of transsexual feelings very early on.

Such individuals may appear for GP help and counsel either physically dressed as a male, or else already cross-dressed as a female and taking 'acquired' female hormones. They often have awareness of available operations and are seeking to be pointed, not to any psychiatric or psychotherapeutic counselling, but to a urological 'transplant' surgeon. If initially not taken too seriously, they may indicate depressive symptoms, talk of taking their own lives, or talk of undertaking self-mutilation in castration. Discussion sometimes reveals that the transsexual has already made efforts to de-sex his masculinity.

Surgeons who undertake the eventual cometic and reconstructive surgery are unlikely to do so until such a patient has undergone psychiatric assessment for a reasonable period. Assuming that psychotherapy does not control or reverse the feminine feelings, and that is usually so, the programme begins with the use of feminizing hormones, depilation of unwanted hair, and attending a speech therapist for voice counselling. This period lasts 18–24 months.

A better chance of success in transition from male to female is assured when ordinary female (XX) companions find they can accept the partially feminized transsexual during the 'trial hormone' period. Also better candidates for success are those who (like the homosexual mentioned earlier) marry and stay married to cover their problem by appearing 'normal'.

Transvestism

Males cross-dressing in women's underclothes and overclothes may be neither transsexuals nor feminine character male homosexuals. They may simply be heterosexuals who enjoy the feeling of women's garments in a passive sexual form or as part of precoital sex play, or simply to relieve a fetishist excitement in relation to female garments. Counselling may be sought by a wife or lady partner who has not been told of the activity by her husband, and who is puzzled, upset, antagonistic or feels degraded and let down by a man. Counselling may be sought by the man himself because he dislikes these feelings and needs, or because he has upset his wife or children on being seen in women's clothes or underwear, for example.

Some transvestites - the condition is a dynamic one - may undertake trips outside the bedroom and home to get the thrill and feel of being taken for a real women. Some progress to extramarital activities in which dressing up as a female is involved. A few may even progress to a professed transsexualism with its wider implications. The pleasure of dressing up as a woman may be turned to profitability by actors and entertainers who make a living from appearing 'in drag'.

Fetishism

This really only becomes a problem when the sexual pleasure and excitement achieved through observing or contact with the fetish object totally replaces the need and desire for sexual intercourse and general heterosexual relationships. This is a difficulty which is not easily overcome with psychotherapy and general counselling. Specialist help from a psychiatrist and clinical psychologist is usually indicated.

There are all degrees of fetish interest, however, in which a sexually stimulating object or objects is desired as an arousal factor, as a foreplay agency, or as part of a continuing sexual stimulation during coitus. The object may be part of the human body - breast, nipple, foot, umbilicus, anus, hairy areas, for example - or it may be an article of clothing - bra, knickers, basque, garters - or it may be material - rubber, silk, transparent nylon - or it may be the colour of the object - black, red, yellow, for example. Leather and rubber items may be part of a sexual foreplay or arousal activity known as 'bondage', or temporary tying up of either partner in a pseudopower play. The items may also feature in sadomasochistic sexual activity as discussed earlier.

Unusual fetish objects seem to feature in the 'correspondence columns' of male oriented magazines, presumably in part because male partners are more fetish users than female partners. Examples include:

amputee fetish
deformity fetish
size fetish (fat and thin in extremes)
skin colour fetish

Counsel is sometimes sought where the lady partner dislikes the use of fetish objects in sexual play, or sees them as a challenge or competition to her own sexual capacities for arousal of her partner.

Swopping and group sex

For some individuals, men or women, the notion of one partner at a time in a heterosexual relationship is not acceptable. It is constraining, irksome, too much like marriage (if the partners are not so), and lacks spice, excitement or appeal in a sexual context. A move to a new environment - housing estate, new town, for example - or move to a new job or move up the social or work ladder, opens up opportunities for new contacts. Mutual personal arousal may offer the 'restricted' partner a chance for extramarital or non-regular partner sexual intercourse, whether at parties, social get-togethers, or within working hours.

In so-called free thinking or liberal sexual partnerships, instead of a new one-to-one relationship, the couple agree with another couple on mutual partner exchange - swopping or wife-swopping or swinging, as it is known. This agreed joint adultery (assuming all parties are married), or partner exchange, may continue only for two couples or be extended to larger groups. Such couple exchanges may be disguised as 'accidental', or openly arranged, or even developed through advertising discreetly in 'contact' magazines.

For married couples, in the long run, swopping or swinging may overtly add new horizons to the sexuality of the partners but covertly offers a specific strain on the marriage itself. Instead of sexual acceptance with partners working out their needs and patterns of mutual pleasure and love, sexual competition and sexual comparisons are being made and activated. The marriage which is already unstable is at greatest risk to swinging or swopping. Jealousy, discrimination, argument, recrimination, loss of loyalty and absence of love may undermine the foundation of even a firm marriage. The risk of sexually transmitted disease is also considerable, the wider the swinging group. Nor is being many years married, protective in holding partners together.

ORGANIC ILLNESS

The significance of organic sources of sexual dysfunction in men is relatively small in early adult life. By middle years , this has increased in importance from the 10% level. Once over 70, degenerative disease as well as acquired illness becomes very relevant and may combine with psychological upset to produce poorly amenable or irreversible sexual disturbance in all phases of coitus.

Organic faults in the sexual apparatus may limit mechanical action or hormonal output, or there may be a combination of both elements. We mentioned penis size earlier and it is true that congenital micropenis may cause problems, in its infantile format. We have also mentioned the 'free floating' penis, with an associative primitive vagina or cloaca, whose proximal end is not connected for nerve or hormonal stimulation to arousal erection.

Inflammation - and the prostate

Inflammation of the penis and scrotum and testicles comes in a variety of presentations, which may create temporary or more chronic sexual dysfunction. Peyronie's inflammation, for example, a fairly uncommon but readily identified chronic inflammatory process, begins in the tunica albuginea and invades the adjacent structures. On arousal and erection, pain occurs as the penis bends dorsally and the man has coital discomfort. Bacterial urethritis and non-specific urethritis can inhibit successful erection because of pain and tension, until suitable chemotherapy is exhibited. Later, if scarring occurs or a stricture develops, ejaculatory upset replaces erectile disturbance. Viral orchitis or bacterial orchitis can also occur, which hopefully clears after therapy or self-healing. Permanent damage means that the testicles may no longer bear sperm and that testosterone may also be depleted.

The prostate is also proximate to the genital apparatus and contributes to the fluid ejaculate. Prostatitis is a well-recognized illness in which aching and discomfort on arousal or near coitus, inhibits first erection holding, then ejaculation.

Diabetic effects - other hormones

The incidence of diabetes mellitus rises with advancing years, so that more that half of all new cases (admittedly mostly non insulin dependent diabetes) are diagnosed after the age of 50. Among the undesirable complications of diabetes mellitus are diabetic neuropathy and autonomic disturbance. Not surprisingly, erectile dysfunction and ejaculatory disorders of organic origin should initiate a search for cryptic disbetes. Where the patient is a known diabetic, a full assessment of the diabetic state - blood glucose on waking and at intervals during the day, glycosuria levels, and glycosylated haemoglobin level - must be undertaken. While restabilization of diabetes is no guarantee of a full reversal of sexual upsets, it can and does contribute to some degree of improvement in many sufferers. (See Table 4.3.)

Classically, in diabetes, failure of erection or upset of ejaculation precedes loss of libido. This view has sometimes been challenged, since sometimes the awareness or discovery by a diabetes sufferer that he may eventually develop sexual difficulties can result in anxiety or depression and supress libido - going on to the very problem originally feared. All degrees of disturbed libido and organic dysfunction are, in fact, possible.

Another hormonal dysfunction which can limit erectile efficiency, both directly by reduced metabolic function and indirectly via reduction in libido, is hypothyroidism. Much less common in men, hypo-thyrodism can occur in early to senior years. The chances of sexual improvement on replacement therapy with thyroxine depend not only on the premorbid libido and sexual capacity but also, in older citizens, on the degree of cerebral and testicular arteriosclerosis which is coincidentally present. In the opposite state of thyrotoxicosis, increased autonomic flow may or may not increase arousal states, but is not likely to increase libido as a rule.

Returning again to diabetes from a different angle, the presence of glycosuria can encourage local penile and urethral infections, balanitis and urethritis, which are persistent until the diabetes is controlled and the infection (fungal or bacterial) is cleared. Coitus may be too painful during the active infection and create temporary dysfunction. This situation may be a feature of the undiagnosed diabetic or of the unstable diabetic, at any age. While younger diabetics may be thin and underweight, older diabetics are often initially markedly overweight. This can add mechanical discomfort in coital positioning. Intertrigo of groins and umbilical area may also be uncomfortable if 'pressed on' during coitus. Weight reduction, better hygiene and local antifungal and anti-inflammatory creams will reverse this mechanical dysfunction problem.

Table 4.3 Sources of sexual dysfunction in diabetes mellitus

Male patients
Anxiety state after awareness of diagnosis
Depression after awareness of diagnosis
Unstable diabetic state -
   hypoglycaemia
   hyperglycaemia
   ketosis
   pre-coma
Peripheral neuropathy
Autonomic dysfunction
Diabetic vascular disease -
   angiopathy
   vasculitis added to arteriosclerosis
Associated illnesses
   thyrotoxicosis
   tuberculosis
Genital and perigenital infections
   balanitis
   urethritis
   intertrigo
   prostatitis
Associative alcoholism
Possible side-effects of drugs
Fear of 'impotence' in intelligent diabetics

Female patients
Anxiety state after awareness of diagnosis
Depression after awareness of diagnosis
Fear of anorgasmia in intelligent diabetics
Unstable diabetic state - as for men
Peripheral neuropathy
Autonomic dysfunction - less clearly evident
Diabetic vascular disease - as for men plus
   reduced clitoral and labial engorgement
   poor or absent orgasm
Associated illnesses
   thyroid excess
   hypothyroidism
   alcoholism
Possible side-effects of drugs

Hypopituitary states are much rarer in men than in women but they can occur - in shock from haemorrhage, in radiation therapy for cerebral or other neoplasm, or from idiopathic cause. The result will be gonadal dysfunction with atrophic changes leading to loss of semen in the ejaculate, lowered male sex hormone levels, but not always a dramatic fall in libido. Secondary sexual hirsutism is lost, a valuable clinical sign. Erectile dysfunction can also appear. Male hormone, thyroxine and steroid hormone replacement therapy given in reverse order may not always correct sexual upset, especially in older men, although hypothyroid and hypoadrenal signs are well reversed. Sometimes more upsetting for the sexually dysfunctional man is the increased feeling of well-being, in turn improving the libido, yet erectile capacity is not restored. In such a case, the male hormone is best withdrawn, leaving thyroxine and fludrocortisone as the substitution or replacement therapy.

Arteriosclerosis

Arteriosclerosis and atheroma are ubiquitous disorders in the blood vessels of all human beings as they age. Nutritional depletion and tissue hypoxia combine to reduce the function of cells, tissues and organs at a variable rate to a variable degree in a given man. The significance of the arteriosclerotic process in sexuality in organic terms can be seen in four areas.

(1)   In the testicular function, advancing arterial degeneration is presumed to discourage sperm production and testosterone release concomitantly. The presumption is a large one, since biopsies do not always coincide with the clinical and sexual findings, and men in their seventies and eighties have been shown to have viable sperm even in their reduced total ejaculate. Measuring the serum testosterone also often fails to confirm the presence of testicular arteriosclerosis since the adrenal glands, if reasonably active, can compensate for lack of male sex hormone from the testes. The presence of a low serum testosterone, alongside declining libido and poor or absent erectile function, may be regarded as the 'male climacteric', especially if accompanied by fatigue, lethargy, mild depression or anxiety. Oral androgen therapy, however, may only improve the sense of wellbeing in the over seventies without restoring erectile capacity, so the assumption of arteriosclerotic change may then be reasonable.

(2)   Cerebral arteriosclerosis, with or without hypertension, can result in diffuse changes in the anterior and middle cortex areas. The resulting organic dementia (or chronic brain syndrome) may

produce loss of libido and loss of erectile capacity, or disinhibition and sexual excitability but still with poor capacity. Inappropriate masturbation, genital exhibition or attempts to 'assault' wife or other women indicate the loss of insight and control. Social and marital disturbance may elicit a need for GP counselling - and the use of tranquillizers or antiandrogen drugs.

(3)   Cerebral infarction or thrombosis, affecting the middle cerebral artery, may result in 'stroke' with variable hemiparesis, plus or minus sensory disturbance, visual or speech disturbance. While libido may be suppressed during the acute and immediate poststroke phases, a resurgence of sexual drive towards premorbid levels can appear. Because of bilateral innervation, 'stroke' does not preclude erection and ejaculation. Attempts at coitus may fail for several reasons. Anxiety on the part of the stroke sufferer may produce psychological block and failure with subsequent fear of failure continuing the problem. Anxiety may also be due to awareness that coitus does raise the blood pressure, and both partners may fear further stroke or complication. Specific counselling as well as drug therapy may be valuable, as we shall discuss later. Organic dysfunction can follow stroke which creates a bilateral pyramidal tract and cortical discorder, i.e. further stroke or strokes on the opposite side to the earlier lesion. Apart from organic and psychological problems, the healthy partner may decline coitus because of a cosmetic or emotional 'turn-off' at the disability of her partner.

(4)   Arteriosclerosis can be significant - with atheroma, in the aortic and iliac vessels of middle years. This, in turn, may deplete the flow to the corpora cavernosa and the penile arteries, even when the neurological and hormonal functions are intact and there is no psychological or emotional problem. This 'vascular insufficiency' may be associated with intermittent claudication of both legs, in middle to senior years. The coming of aortic and large vessel grafts for obliterative aerterial illness may also resolve erectile problems of vascular origin. We should note that the simpler expedient of bilateral lumbar sympathectomy, may improve blood flow but rob the man of neurological control of erection or, more specifically, ejaculation.

Parkinsonism - and dopamine

The clinical syndrome of tremor, rigidity and bradykinesia spells out parkinsonism with a frequency of one patient in 100 over 60 years of age (and one in 1000 in younger years). The features of this complaint would indicate likely mechanical problems in sexual intercourse, because of the stiffness, shaking and slow movements of not just the limbs but the face and trunk. Before chemotherapy became available, medical observers had noted not just mechanical problems in such patients but a clear decline or loss in libido, with secondary erectile dysfunction.

The introduction of dopamine in the late 1960s proved a boon to those suffering from degenerative parkinsonism, in whom dopamine depletion had been identified as a 'neurotransmitter problem'. Patients in whom parkinsonism was associated with cerebral arteriosclerosis, or who had postencephalitic forms, or who were head-injury induced sufferers, were less likely to benefit, in theory at least, from dopamine replacement therapy.

The recovery of physical control and function with dopamine was often noticeably accompanied by a resurgence of libido and improved erectile function. This was not a matter of 'aphrodisiac therapy', since those with a previous low libido or erectile problem prior to the onset of parkinsonism did not show such changes. Patients with milder forms of parkinsonism may be treated initially with anticholinergic drugs. As a side-effect, however, such drugs may aggravate erectile difficulties which have already appeared, and this possibility has to be kept in mind. Bromocriptine, as an alternative antiparkinson drug, occasionally encourages increased libido or erectile improvement, not only because it is a dopamine agonist but also because it reduces a high serum prolactin.

Vascular illness apart, disease and degeneration of the central nervous system can affect erectile and ejaculatory function. This may be the result of accidental, or deliberate, trauma affecting the discs, the vertebrae or the pelvic bones. Brain injury may be severe and either create loss of libido or loss of arousal capacity. In disc prolapse, pain may interfere with libido and mechanical capacity. In cord compression due to cervical spondylosis, lower limb weakness and sphincter disturbance in middle to senior years can be associated with loss of erectile and ejaculatory function.

Trauma to the spinal cord, resulting in its being cut completely above the first lumbar level, still leaves the male coital reflex available. Erection can be provoked by contact stimulation in the genital and perigenital areas. A skilled lady partner can actively capture the penis erect in her vagina, and stimulate further to orgasm. Partial cut of the cord by trauma creates marked lower limb spasticity. This offers, like the situation in sex for congenital spastic individuals, mechanical problems in coital positioning and entry.

In the cord demyelination of multiple sclerosis, any nerve groups can be made dysfunctional or nonoperational as a transient or, later, permanent phenomenen. It should not be overlooked that the emotional and anxiety problems of multiple sclerosis sufferers can induce psychological erectile upset. As with diabetes, libido may be well maintained in the face of a range of dysfunctions, from poor erection, to failed ejaculation, to loss of orgasmic sensation altogether. Sphincter control problems are sometimes an additional burden for the male partner.

Venereal diseases - operations

Sexually transmitted disease can also produce organic problems in relation to erection and ejaculation. Gonococcal and non-specific urethritis have already been noted as temporary inhibitors of the mechanics of coitus. Postgonococcal urethral stricture may produce ejaculatory upset. The return of syphilis to the venereal scene in the 1970s and onwards accounts for current and prospective loss of erectile function as part of the symptomatology of tabes dorsalis (locomotor ataxy). This should not be a feature of those whose primary infection was effectively treated by organism-sensitive antibiotics. Acquired immune deficiency syndrome, and some cases of infective hepatitis, are acquired through sexual contact. The active illness produces severe lethargy, fatigue and system problems but it is the fall off in libido that accounts for any sexual dysfunction as a general rule.

Operative therapy, as we have earlier noted, can induce psychological block with secondary erectile dysfunction. The operation of prostatectomy is traditionally associated in the lay mind with secondary loss of male potency. Yet contemporary transurethral (not open) prostatectomy should not affect the power of erection if it was previously satisfactory. Where there was a problem, organic, emotional or mixed, then postoperative anxiety is likely to interfere with successful arousal and erection. Variable problems can arise from organic upset, however, in relation to ejaculation after prostate resection. Resection of the bladder neck may result in flow incompetence so that the ejaculation becomes retrograde, not antegrade. When sexual intercourse is resumed about 4–6 weeks postoperatively, the man and his lady partner may be surprised at the impaired ejaculate, and will need effective reassurance that otherwise all is well.

Any operation may be followed by reduction in libido, or by anxiety which leads to emotional block and dysfunction. The operations around the lower abdomen and pelvis may have no genital link at all, but lack of information and lack of positive counsel can induce psychological erectile disorder. Preoperative counsel is best.

Arthritis - and other system diseases

Arthritis can appear at any time of life, not merely in senior years. Joint disorders of inflammatory origin can give pain and stifness, and reduced agility, which interfere with the positional and activity mechanics of coitus. The older individual is likely to have varying degrees of lumbosacral, hips or knees osteoarthritis, for example, which may discourage efforts at sexual intercourse. Sometimes patients learn by themselves how to utilize more comfortable positioning, or to take precoital analgesics, or have a warm bath prior to coitus, in order to be at peak 'fitness' for the sexual pleasure. Patients who have had hip replacement and are sexually active, may comment on the new lease of sexual as well as social and working life afforded to them. Severe disability from rheumatoid arthritis may involve counselling on 'alternative' sexual pleasuring, where regular coitus is precluded.

Coronary artery disease, and myocardial ischaemia and failure, remain a major health problem of affluent societies. Advice may be sought on the safety or risks of coitus in cardiac patients: those with angina, with recent myocardial infarction, with controlled congestive heart failure, and after coronary artery bypass. Patients not so counselled may report loss of libido from anxiety, fear, chest pain, breathlessness, or associative emotional erectile dysfunction. Good coronary care departments and coronary bypass units offer specific advice on sexual activity to the patient and partner which may, or may not, resolve or prevent problems.

Organic loss of erectile function in coronary artery disease is unlikely to occur, unless the illness is part of severe widespread atherosclerosis or unless it is induced by the drugs used in treating the myocardial ischaemia or failure.

Chronic obstructive airways disease may cause difficulties in relation to the physiological need for increase in respiratory rate, during the arousal to orgasmic phases of coitus. Severe dyspnoea induced by sexual activity may create a conscious decision to avoid coitus. Fear of aggravating the chronic lung disorder may produce psychological erectile dysfunction. Bronchospasm may be part of the chronic obstructive airways scene, or it can be present as bronchial asthma alone. Emotional stress and excitement can be asthma triggers, and there are asthmatic patients whose wheezing and dyspnoea are induced by coital activity or even by masturbatory action. Sometimes, what appears to be sex-exercise-induced asthma proves to be related to the environmental site of coital activity. Dusts, feathers, house mites or, for example, bedclothes are the real trigger agencies - allergic asthma rather than emotional or autonomic agency asthma.

Patients with chronic renal failure are often in the young to middle years group, and have been sexually active. Mechanical or peritoneal dialysis is keeping them reasonably active, in many cases until a kidney is available for permanent relief if possible. The anxiety and stress of the need for regular dialysis may depress libido. Drug immuno-suppression may have a part in this as well. In some uraemic patients, erectile dysfunction is related to a rise in serum prolactin. In others, reduced spermatogenesis and reduced serum testosterone are contri-butory agencies. The paradoxical aspect in sexual terms is that libido and function are failing, while the general health is at least partially improved on the dialysis programme.

Rheumatic diseases affecting younger citizens, rheumatoid arthritis and ankylosing spondylitis in particular, have frequently affected activities of daily living. Reduced range of joint movements, painful sensations, tiredness and fatigue all combine to handicap the young man or woman. We might anticipate libido and sexual enjoyment would be reduced. In relation to partners, we might picture that mutual satisfaction would be reduced as well. All the studies of sexuality and rheumatoid diseases indicate that feelings of love and caring in a stable happy partnership (marital or not) will overcome many of the difficulties that sexology had anticipated. While joint restrictions may seem obvious - and in ankylosing spondylitis, back movement limitations - the muscular energy required for coitus would seem to be a restricting factor. Fatigue is a key depressant in relation to sexuality in any illness. How much more likely in rheumatoid diseases that inhibit musculoskeletal health.

Back pain is often thought of as a limiting factor in the sexuality of women. It may be just as relevant in male sexuality. Physiotherapy departments treating male back pain do not usually enquire about the sexual drive and sexual activity of their attenders, unless this information is, of course, volunteered. Yet several studies suggest that recent loss of libido may be a positive element in backache, especially where there is no neuropathic pathology. In other words, where the patient, male or female, comes to the doctor with a complaint of backache, it is appropriate to make tactful enquiries about sexual drive, sexual interest and sexual patterns of outlet. Backache may produce not just pain as a limiting mechanical factor but anxiety and tension to augment any sexual dysfunction. This in turn implies that conventional analgesia - tablets, heat, massage, surgical support - is insufficient if a sexual problem is extant. Psychotherapy is also required.

MENTAL ILLNESS

To some extent, the relationship between sexual illness and sexuality may be seen as a two way process. For example, anxiety neurosis and endogenous depression may contain in their presentation a decline or loss of libido and erectile or ejaculatory dysfunction. The tension or gloom is presumed to dampen cortical arousal mechanisms or inhibit corticospinal flow to the genital organs. Oppositely, however, the appearance of erectile or ejaculatory difficulties in a previously mentally fit man can result in anxiety states or reactive depression. At times it may be difficult to see which came first - the faulty function or the anxiety or depression.

Anxiety - and depression

In preceding parts of this book, we have considered a variety of effects on sexual drive and capacity in relation to mental illness. Anxiety states may be induced by environmental upset, bereavement, divorce, departure of partner, illness in a loved one, personal organic illness, or for no clear and overt reason at all. The fears, tremblings, hyperpnoea and somatic symptoms of all kinds may be accompanied by libido decline, erectile dysfunction and failure. Phobic states are another example of anxiety illness and may, as we have noted, include sexual problems from aversion as well as loss of libido. Anxiety may also be linked with obsessive compulsive disorder. In such patients, sexual difficulties may arise because of, for example, cleansing rituals before, during or after sexual intercourse, or because of disturbing repetitive acts which delay intercourse. The need to use drugs in any of the anxiety forms may, in turn, exacerbate libido or erectile dysfunction. On the other hand, psychotherapy and drug control of the anxiety states may permit sexual drive and sexual capacity to improve. Disorders of affect symptoms can include sexual dysfunction, as we have also considered earlier. Depression may occur alone, or as part of an anxiety depression, or as part of biopolar disturbance, i.e. manic depressive illness. Sometimes these affective disorders may seem to start off as an extension of recognizable sadness or elation in response to circumstance - loss, happy surprise, as in bereavement or childbirth - but more often the affective upset is not linked with any regular pattern and is more filled out and distinct in essence.

The characteristics of depression include withdrawal from loving and physical interpersonal exchange, and decline in emotional ties, moving away from happiness to feelings of guilt and unworthiness and considerations of death. All these impair libido and encourage erectile failure.

The features of mania, whose expression may vary from milder hypomanic states to florid disorientation, delusions and hallucinations, include euphoria, insomnia, apparently limitless energy, expressions of grandiosity and low frustration tolerance. The results in sexual terms may be similar to those of depression, with loss of libido and decreased sexual capacity. Occasionally, the hypomanic individual shows increased sexual drive, makes increased sexual demands and refuses to be turned away for legitimate or other reasons put forward by the partner.

Schizophrenia presents us with a wider range of sexual patterns. The aetiology remains unsure. The individual may be withdrawn and 'cut off' in behaviour and indulge in no coital efforts or interpersonal sexual contact. Such 'loners' do sometimes masturbate as if some sexual relief is still needed. Occasionally the schizophrenic patient shows signs of excessive sexual interest and eagerness for sexual outlet. Thirdly, the schizophrenic may show inappropriate sexual behaviour towards carers, hospital staff, visitors or others.

Pre-senile dementia

The other major mental illness, organic dememtia, has already been considered. It should be recalled that in addition to arteriosclerosis producing chronic brain failure, the condition may appear in old and younger individuals as part of Alzheimer's disease, or as part of Huntington's chorea later in the illness. Loss of memory, especially for recent events, emotional lability, and intellectual changes are classical features of dementia. Libido may be lost or may be reportedly increased but even in the latter case, the sexual behaviour known to occur is usually inappropriate in open company, efforts at seduction in the wrong place with the wrong person, may all take place. Efforts at voyeurism may cause relatives more distress. Efforts at homosexual contact in a man who has always apparently had heterosexual drive are sometimes seen. This may indicate latent suppressed homosexuality, now disinhibited, or simply be a deviation induced by loss of mental insight. Any of these inappropriate sexual acts may bring the man into unintended contact with the law.

Hysterical neurosis, or conversion disorder, implies an upset of function in the nervous system not explained by identifiable organic lesions. These may be motor or sensory in character. Erectile or ejaculatory dysfunction is not usually listed as a feature in this disorder yet it may well be so in some patients. The factors of primary and secondary gain may apply, particularly in the presence of marital or interpersonal problems. Such individuals may be anxious, irritable or depressed as an adjunctive factor in the sexual dysfunction. The personality may be a histrionic one or even an antisocial one. Such patients may be able to erect the penis satisfactorily but fail to ejaculate as desired.

DRUGS

Medication and drugs in general may have an adverse or a positive effect on human sexuality. In this section we shall consider the adverse effects of drugs - taken alone or in combination, on the prescription of doctors or in the way of self-prescription. It is worth noting that patients may sometimes blame their medication, to account for loss of libido or erectile difficulties, when there is no record of a possible link between the action and side-effects of the medication and problems of a sexual nature. Oppositely, patients may swear by the effectiveness of a medication - paracetamol, vitamin C, yeast, vitamin E - in restoring or improving libido or erectile capacity, and be unwilling to acknowledge the likely placebo effect.

Some drugs will be recognized in advance as likely to depress libido, suppress male sex hormone effects, and interfere with male potency in coitus. In prostatic carcinoma, for example, drug therapy even with the currently lower doses of stilboestrol is likely to lower libido and create erectile dysfunction if this is not already extant. The alternative chemotherapy using the antiandrogen, cyproterone acetate, is likewise a suppressive to male libido and will effectively create lack of arousal and erection. This antiandrogen drug is actively used in some cases of antisocial sexuality, for example, in dementia or in hypersexuality syndromes, to suppress male libido and control the individual behaviour.

A long recognized more familiar group of drugs known to interfere in male sexuality are those used to treat essential or other forms of hypertension. The very early drugs like reserpine affected human sexuality by depleting amines as a central action. Later medication, with drugs that interfered directly with autonomic blood pressure control, were almost bound to cause male sexual difficulties.

Hypotensives and thymoleptics

The original ganglion blockers produced erectile and ejaculatory dysfunction. The current selective β-blockers can still cause problems, more usually with ejaculation than with erection. The first line therapy in mild hypertension is still thiazide diuretics but they too may affect erectile function. The newer generation of hypotensive agents aims at reducing blood pressure by vasodilation. Prazosin, for example, is an α-blocker but with vasodilator properties and nifedipine is a calcium antagonist with vasodilator properties. In theory, vasodilation should encourage erectile capacity and may indeed do so, provided the blood pressure does not fall too much. Excessive vasodilation has an occasional risk of inducing a type of priapism, with hydralazine and prazosin both reported in this respect. This possibility potentially increases if the patient has an unrecognized degree of congestive cardiac failure. ACE inhibitors can be used then, instead.

In the treatment of affective disorder, depression can and does respond to tricyclic and tetracyclic drugs which are thymoleptic. Since depression, as we noted earlier, is invariably associated with depressed libido and erectile upsets, we should expect the thymoleptics to restore the picture to premorbid levels. This may begin to occur, only for the medication to reverse the excellent trend by encouraging a rise in serum prolactin levels. This in turn has an antiandrogenic effect. Testicular swelling and gynaecomastia may be accompanying signs of the problem.

Where the tranquillizers are used to control anxiety - diazepam or oxazepam, for example - the beneficial effects may be offset by a central effect on libido. This is another reason for the general advice to use these agents for short periods only, and to add psychotherapy as direct treatment.

H2 Antagonists - and others

The H2 antagonists have rightly been welcomed in the therapy and healing of peptic ulceration. Cimetidine has been available much longer than its nearest rival, ranitidine. Reports of erectile dysfunction in men treated with cimetidine have been linked to two features of the drug. It may induce raised prolactin levels, as witness the appearance of gynaecomastia or it may interfere with cerebral H2 receptors. The effects are, in part, dose related but may also represent an individual sensitivity since clearly not every patient on H2 antagonists reports the occurence of sexual problems - in fact, relatively small numbers only at the time of writing. Any such case reported must therefore be looked at in terms of psychological as well as possible organic sources. Using ranitidine as an alternative may also be worth a trial but bear in mind that this drug too might act centrally on H2 receptors. Curiously, cimetidine has been shown to lower male sperm count yet reportedly raise serum testosterone levels.

In chemotherapy by cytotoxic and alkylating drugs, there is a risk of peripheral neuropathy and autonomic neuropathy as side-effects, among many others. First, the seriously debilitating nature of much neoplastic disease may cause reduced physical and muscular capacity, and the anxiety or depression about the diagnosis and therapy may suppress libido. Then the neuropathies may exacerbate or underscore the loss of erectile and ejaculatory capacities. Vincristine is particularly likely to produce the last named. Cyclophosphamide can induce testicular atrophic changes. Such side-effects are important to recall when counselling a male patient undergoing therapy.

The diuretic and potassium sparing chemical, spironolactone, as well as the cardiac efficiency-improving chemical, digitalis, may both interfere sometimes with erectile capacity. Gynaecomastia may appear in association with such sexual disturbances.

A high serum prolactin in women may cause scanty or absent menses, loss of vaginal lubricity and secondary dyspareunia. In addition, sexual interest may also fall. In men, high serum prolactin also may depress sexual interest. More specifically, there is erectile dysfunction and a drop in the sperm count. In both sexes, many neurotransmitters affect prolactin secretion so that any medication which inhibits, say, dopamine action can, in turn, raise serum prolactin levels. The antinauseant drug, metoclopramide (also used in peptic ulcer and migraine) can do this, as can the antianxiety family of phenothiazines like promazine and chlorpromazine. Another drug used in mental health problems, the antihallucinant, pimozide, can likewise raise serum prolactin. Such patients may already have poor libido and sex dysfunction because of the schizoid or schizophrenic illness itself. Pimozide then compounds the sexual problem although effective against the other features of the illness.

In relation to users of female sex hormones, as a birth control mechanism or for problems of a noncontraceptive nature, we should not overlook the fact that oestrogens can raise serum prolactin levels through the governor action on the anterior pituitary. However, there is no fixed response in this connection. In some patients, a particular drug may be blamed for causing a rise in serum prolactin and thereby influencing sexuality. Again, however, we should be circumspect about such reports. Anxiety and stress alone can excite the cortical, hypothalamic and anterior pituitary linkages and thereby encourage a raised prolactin level in the serum. The other trigger factor, more erotic in character, is derived from caressing and sucking or nipping the nipples in sexual foreplay or play.

Drugs which induce depression can in turn affect libido with reports of secondary dysfunction. Such medications include clonidine and methyldopa, as well as the already mentioned reserpine. They also include indomethacin and the corticosteroids and both levodopa and the phenothiazines. The popularly used supportive drug of obesity control, fenfluramine, may sometimes be followed by depression after its routine withdrawal.

Alcohol

Although not considered as a drug in any therapeutic sense, all forms of alcohol are used to enhance a feeling of wellbeing, ease anxiety and stress, improve socializing in group situations, act as a sedative or nightcap, and augment the pleasure of social occasions like meals out, parties and weddings. In men who have sexual anxiety for one reason or another, alcohol may be taken deliberately when the possibility of coitus looms close upon the partnership horizon. In the man who is not an alcoholic, there is a fine balance between the disinhibition in sexual behaviour which alcohol may induce, and the loss of erectile capacity or rapid falling away of erection achieved (detumescence or else premature ejaculation). Hence the traditional and often true saying that alcohol improves the sexual drive and arousal but is likely to decrease the success of performance.

Alcohol in excess, and especially in psychopathic or emotionally unstable individuals, may encourage antisocial and aggressive sexual acts. These include exhibitionism, indecent assault, rape and anal sex. The element of aggression and assault with violence may be increased if the man is frustrated by his alcohol-induced loss of erectile potency.

In any case, once alcohol has induced loss of erection, the fear of failure may take over as a psychological block even if further intake of alcohol is avoided. Alcohol may also cause problems because it can light up a latent prostatitis in adult and older men. Under the influence of alcohol, too, a man who would otherwise not have exposed himself to the risk of venereal infection, may do so and subsequently develop the sexual problems of organic origin already considered.

The heavy drinker and the confirmed alcoholic can develop cirrhosis of the liver. Excess oestrogen effects - most commonly seen clinically in the form of gynaecomastia, spider naevi and pink palms - can encourage loss of erectile capacity as well. Oedema and excess aldosterone in the blood may be treated in cirrhosis by using spironolactone, a drug which we have already noted may be associated with loss of male potency. Another effect of alcoholism and poor nutrition is the development of peripheral neuropathy. This can further add to problems of erectile control.

Various therapeutic approaches to alcoholism include psychotherapy, group therapy (Alcoholics Anonymous) and the use of aversion therapy. The latter may utilize the drug, disulfiram, quite effectively. Erectile dysfunction has, it should be noted, been blamed on the action of disulfiram, although care needs to be taken in apportioning blame as a side-effect in any given patient. Sexual activity does need healthy muscles, healthy metabolic function and good exercise capacity. The severe alcoholic is often undernourished or underweight and so his fitness for the gymnastics of sexuality is often in doubt, or simply not present at all. This is perhaps more obvious in the alcoholic man who is over 60 years old, or who has concomitant problems in other body systems, such as anaemia or chronic obstructive airways disease.

Alcohol is also responsible for inducing depression in heavy and regular users. This may add further to erectile and ejaculation difficulties.

The alcohol user may also be a user of clandestine, illegal drugs or drugs of dependency. Cocaine, hashish, mescaline, lysergic acid, amphetamines, barbiturates, azepam drugs and the opiates are taken for many reasons. Among these is often included the claim that they enhance sexual experience, prolong sexual performance, raise arousal levels, improve erectile capacity and reverse any sexual difficulties. Doctors need no spelling out of the risk to brain and other body systems which such drug abuse may evolve. Long-term usage is more likely to discourage erectile function, and that includes hashish, widely claimed by users to be less harmful than alcohol. In 'beginner' users, any apparent aphrodisiac effect is derived from the mood, wishes and eagerness of the partners and not from any true stimulant to the contributory systems of coitus.

Alcoholism, with or without drug abuse, can also produce a dementia which in turn depresses libido and erectile capacity. In senior citizens, it is not always easy to distinguish the alcohol effects from those of arteriosclerosis. Sadly, even if the alcoholism is brought under control, there is no guarantee of full reversal of the dementia or of the sexuality deficiencies. Studies of alcoholics as a general group suggest that chronic fatigue and tiredness, with or without depressive elements, also contribute to reduced sexual drive and later reduced sexual outlet. In the early months to years of alcoholism, it is a change in quality rather than in quantity (frequency) which is reported - at least until total erectile dysfunction arrives in the picture.

5
Common Sexual Problems in the Female Partner

The problems of erection and ejaculation in the male partner clearly have no direct analogy in the female partner. Sexual desire, and sexual arousal, and orgasm are the three elements in which difficulties and dysfunction may be seen. Considering the research and investigations that have gone on for so many years into male problems, it is not surprising that the information, studies and understanding of female problems has lagged so far behind - at least until the coming of women's liberation movements and the strive for sexual equality in personal relationships and within the marriage setting. Even so, the development of birth control, of family planning clinics and of antenatal and postnatal care, inevitably and often starkly highlighted many areas of sexual difficulty in women attending for such contraception. They also indirectly threw into perspective many of the male problems as well.

ALTERED LIBIDO

The original work of Kinsey and his co-workers reported at the end of the 1940s, suggested that, taken overall, libido and sexual interest peaked in the third decade of life, in contrast to the male peaks in the late teens and early twenties. In an earlier chapter, we looked at several of the factors which affect the pattern of sexual drive in both sexes. Kinsey's work suggested an age influence. Studies in England of the sexual behaviour of women after 50 noted that, the pressures of society and the focal problems of the menopause notwithstanding, older women with suitable partners can continue to have active sex lives. In some, maturity and overcoming of earlier inhibitions permit more enjoyment and pleasure so that libido may rise rather than fall away. May Duddle of Manchester has stated, however, there is some evidence that more women than men tend to lose desire to join in sexual activities in middle to senior years.

Since libido in women is just as dynamic and subject to fluctuation as it is in men, we should hardly be surprised at the variety of psychological, emotional and physical agencies which can alter its intensity. Consideration of the physiological states of womanhood - the menstrual cycle, pregnancy, lactation, the menopause - in the healthy subject might indicate even greater likelihood of libido alterations and variations. We should not forget, however, that androgens play a part in initiating and enhancing desire or appetite for sex and, in turn, a need for sexual outlet. Biology might suggest that peak sexual desire should occur in and around the ovulatory phase of the menstrual cycle. At that point, androgens may be taking over from the high oestrogen level. Thereafter the influence of progesterone and the appearance of premenstrual tension syndrome may lower the libido from its alleged high point.

There are still no satisfactory studies which can marry up neatly and invariably the hormonal levels and the behaviour patterns of libido to give predictability in a given woman. The situation is no clearer for those women whose natural menstrual cycle control is modified by the use of steroidal oral contraceptives. The changes in sexual drive and sexual responsiveness of women on the contraceptive pill may be obvious or subtle, may be positive or negative, may be reported or unreported but are nowhere consistent overall.

Altered libido is sometimes classified under two 'working labels' which at first sight seem almost identical. These are:

Inadequate arousal
Inadequate arousability

The former condition refers to the woman who reports no great regular sexual interest or desire. She can, however, be aroused and may even enjoy full orgasmic expression. The latter state covers absent interest and desire, and no response under any circumstance.

In Table 5.1 we can see a comprehensive list of psychological and organic factors which may alter libido in a negative direction. Clearly these may occur as individual elements or in any combination within, or across, the two main categories.

Anxiety state or anxiety neurosis may be an ongoing personality problem, or may arise in relation to short-term environmental circumstances. Some women cope better with work demands, family crises, money problems, interim illness, for example, than others.

Table 5.1 Factors altering libido in women. Possible negative agencies

Psychological:	Anxiety state
	Depression
	Non-sexual marital friction
	Fear of aggression or assault
	Fear of pain
	Fear of pregnancy
	Fear of infection
	Performance anxiety
	Fear of discovery (pre and extramarital)
	Partner turn-offs, e.g. cosmetic hygiene ageing illness
	Aversion
	Psychotic illness
	Religious 'guilt'
	Anxieties in pregnancy
	Menopausal upset
	Premenstrual tension
	Vaginismus
Organic:	Local genital infection
	Local scarring
	Drug-induced including 'the pill'
	Physical ill health
	Diabetes mellitus
	Endocrinopathy
	Menopausal upset - vaginal atrophy
	Cervico-uterine disorders
	Postnatal disorders
	Breast feeding

Raised levels of tension either depress sexual drive, or create distraction to the otherwise pleasurable and relaxed situation of physical contact. Occasionally, and oppositely, the anxiety of the environment may lead to sexual vulnerability and transferred libido, if the helper or guide, doctor or not, is a male subject. The women with anxiety and loss of libido may be helped by tranquillizers in the short term, by empathy, by psychotherapy, and by help in restructuring the life problem if possible.

Anxiety may transfer itself, or be part of the scene, in the male partner. We may then be presented with an anxious woman whose sex interest is low, and an anxious man with psychological erectile dysfunction. In that case, there is little use treating and counselling one partner and not the other.

As with features of depression in men, so the signs and symptoms in women - insomnia, apathy, guilt feelings, self neglect, self-reproach, crying - also include a falling away of the libido. When this depression coincides with a woman in the postpartum condition, the male partner may be bewildered by all the changes. From a nuclear family to a three-part family, from keenness to have sexual intercourse to sexual rejection, from being the centre of love and attention to playing second fiddle to the new infant arrival.

When the depression coincides with the menopause, so-called involutional depression, the features are more of agitation and anxiety with a sense of apprehension and are sometimes linked with the idea of loss of femininity (conception is no longer possible within the sexual act). The additional fear of growing old, or of being rejected by the partner in favour of a younger companion, also looms. The opposite pattern is sometimes reported, in which there is a rise or surge in libido, partly because pregnancy is no longer a risk and partly because the woman is testing her continuing sexual attraction for her regular partner. Loss of libido and risk of severe depression with suicide are said to be greater in brighter women, those with advanced education or skills, and ambition or marked drive in earlier years.

In bipolar depression, when the individual shifts to the hypomanic end of the spectrum, a sense of excitement and elation may superficially hint at increased sexual drive and sexual interest. A restless state and inability to relax and concentrate on the pleasure of sexual contact may discount the apparent increase in libido and, indeed, increase any sexual problems that have arisen within the regular relationship.

At least one study, conducted at general practice level in the United Kingdom, reported that 'some patients have an increased interest in sex when depressed' and this phenomenon is 'proportionately more so in females than in males'. The same study showed that two fifths of the patients looked at, either ceased to engage in sexual intercourse or had less frequent coitus. Increased orgasmic difficulty was a feature of some of the depressed women, but much less than the 69% of depressed men who had erectile or ejaculatory dysfunction. Clear loss of libido was noted by one depressed woman in every four studied.

NON-SEXUAL MARITAL PATHOLOGIES

Marriage guidance counsellors are familiar with a whole range of problems which can be described as non-sexual marital friction. These may be money problems - unemployment, redundancy, low wage, being kept short of funds by the husband, conflict over two incomes, excessive spending on drink, gambling, clothes, for example. They may be environmental problems - poor accommodation, house too small, lack of amenities, difficult neighbours, for example. They may be family problems - hyperactive child, mental or physical handicap in a child, lack of friends, betrayal by friends, dislike of husband's friends, interference by relatives including the in-laws, for example. There may be dislike of husband's language, attitude to the home, lack of responsibility and his need to work away from home a good deal. The husband may be possessive, jealous, physically aggressive, verbally aggressive or both.

These are all examples of marital pathology and are more likely to appear, as Jack Dominian has differentiated them, in the 'unhappily married' compared with the 'happily married'. The characteristics of the happily married, he explains, are emotionally stable, considerate of others, yielding, companionable, self-confident, emotionally dependent. By contrast, the unhappily married are emotionally unstable, critical of others, dominating, isolated, lack self-confidence and are emotionally self-sufficient.

Not just altered libido but a whole range of sexual difficulties are more likely in the friction-prone 'unhappily married' partners, the woman and the man alike. There is good argument for the doctor, faced initially with such a couple asking for help with the sexual problems, to refer them initially for marital help from the local marriage guidance service. Either after or during the later stages of such marriage guidance, the specific sexual troubles can be taken up and helped by the medical counsellor.

VIOLENCE AND AGGRESSION

A previously satisfactory libido (or a low level of sexual desire *ab initio*) can be disturbed by an undue content of violence, or aggression of a physical nature. This can present itself under the following circumstances:

Having witnessed an assault or violence in relation to sex in the parental home, of father towards mother.

Having been a childhood victim of sexual assault by male parent or male sibling, or other male outside the family setting.

Having been an adult victim of sexual assault or aggression, whether rape or indecent assault or buggery.

Having experienced sexual demands from her male partner, which involved aggression or the implication of aggression, such as bondage, shackling, flagellation.

Having seen films or video plays involving sexual assault and developed a secondary phobia. A similar phobia may derive from reading the news reports of such incidents.

Having to receive sexual attention with her partner under the influence of alcohol, and thereby being rough and insensitive in love-making.

Having experienced intramarital 'rape', after refusing to have intercourse for one reason or another.

Having participated in drug taking sessions which have culminated in aggressive sexual encounter.

Mental and physical and sexual disturbances that may follow rape have resulted in the setting up of support groups and 'rape crisis centres'. Family doctors are not infrequently asked for help and guidance in any of the circumstances described in the list above. Childhood experiences may have been suppressed, and only re-emerge in the light of marriage and efforts at coitus. Only in the last few years has the incidence of incest and assault and pederasty been revealed as much greater than we have previously considered in our Western society.

DYSPAREUNIA

Biting, pinching, slapping and even scratching may all be a part of enthusiastic foreplay and orgasmic action by either partner. The experience of marked pain, or severe discomfort, at or during intromission of the penis into the vagina, is likely to act as a major 'turnoff' in the otherwise pleasureable experience of the sexual act.

When such pain is repeated, the fear of painful intercourse - more formally called dyspareunia - becomes a depressant agent on the libido. Organic and emotional factors, separately or in combination, may contribute to dyspareunia, and establish the vicious circle of pain-fear-more pain-more fear, and so on.

Causes of dyspareunia (excluding the phenomenon of vaginismus) include the factors shown in Table 5.2.

Table 5.2 Causes of dyspareunia

Light or superficial discomfort	postmenopausal dryness
	local scar tissue after
	    episiotomy or pelvic
	    operation
	local infection of
	    vulva or vagina
	Bartholins abscess
	local anatomical disturbance
	    congenital or
	    acquired

Marked or deep discomfort	endometriosis
	persistent pelvic infection
	cervical ulceration
	intact hymen with haematocolpos
	retroverted uterus
	ovarian prolapse
	osteoarthritis of hips
	osteoarthritis of lumbosacral
	    spine
	carcinoma of vulva, vagina or
	    cervix
	occasionally fibroids

When fear of pain depresses libido and arousal, then, for example, premenstrual lack of lubrication may compound the original cause of dyspareunia. We should recall that one episode of pain may be used as a 'reasonable excuse' against coitus by the woman who has 'turned off' her partner.

The pain may occur outside the pelvic area. For example, angina pectoris can be induced in the ischaemic woman during coital activity. Unless she is instructed on the prophylactic use of glyceryl trinitrate or calcium antagonists or ß-blockers, fear of provoking chest pain may suppress libido sharply. The pain may be in the form of true sexual headache or 'benign orgasmic cephalgia', in which even mild coital activities provokes a bilateral aching or throbbing sensation, involving neck and facial areas as well. Headache from more significant organic sources - arterio-venous malformation, angioma or intracerebral tumour - can also be provoked by coital activity. The latter are more likely to have associative symptoms - ataxy, nausea, vomiting, photophobia, for example - than the 'pure' sexual headache.

Within the pelvic area, inflammation of the bladder either as full-blown cystitis or low-grade recurrent cystitis, can be a source of fear of pain. Sexual activity may light up pain in the joints of patients with chronic rheumatoid disorder or with systemic lupus erythematosus. Patients with the 'frozen shoulder' syndrome, a condition lasting up to

18 months if untreated, may experience lowered libido. Rheumatoid patients have sometimes a painful sternum as part of the syndrome, creating pain in the 'man-over-woman' position, or even side-to-side.

Undoubtedly pain may become established at cerebral level long after the original problem has apparently resolved. The woman may resist this notion of 'fixed pain' in relation to coitus, and require considerable psychotherapy to achieve resolution of her problem.

PREGNANCY

Fear of pregnancy should, in theory at least, have been largely eliminated by the advent of proper family planning and antenatal and postnatal care. Those who wish to enjoy a sexual relationship within or outside marriage can feel free to do so, protected by the hormonal contraceptive pill or by a suitable intravaginal or intrauterine device or, when a planned family has been completed, by sterilization or the partner's vasectomy. This picture is very far from universal. Religious beliefs may preclude using any mechanical or chemical contraceptive. Ignorance of birth control methods still abounds in the shy, embarrassed, indolent, scared or other dominated woman. She may be forced to 'rely on' the male partner's use of a condom or the so-called 'rhythm method' or the still surprisingly frequent withdrawal just prior to ejaculation by the man, coitus interruptus. Partially disabled or handicapped citizens may be at risk because of unwillingness to attend, or inability to visit, the doctor.

The unprotected or 'exposed' woman may have been enjoying a good relationship with her male companion, only to have the seed of doubt implanted at the risks of human seeds being implanted. Such anxiety will certainly reduce the pleasure and excitement of the act and, in time, affect sexual interest and sexual desire. Fear of pregnancy may be exacerbated where the lady partner has gone through a first pregnancy with marked difficulties - severe morning sickness, much heaviness and varicose veins, micturition problems, raised blood pressure, and ultimately difficulties at labour or the birth itself. Such reluctance to re-expose herself to the risk of conception may 'turn off' the mother for a prolonged period after childbirth. This in turn may place not just the sexual relationship but the entire marriage in jeopardy.

INFECTION

While the appearance of the current AIDS virus has made the

homosexual man more circumspect about coitus with more than one homosexual partner on a regular basis, fear of other forms of sexually transmitted infection seems to have played only a minimal part in affecting libido, in men or women. The advent of effective antibiotics and chemotherapy for most forms of genitourinary sexually transmitted illness was, in fact, an agency of encouragement in the climate of sexual freedom that grew in the heterosexual community from the late 1950s onward. Indeed, entertainment stars and other famous members of the 'youth in revolt' generations were almost inclined to wear their exposure to gonorrhoea, for example, as a badge of sexual pride.

There appear to be five circumstances where fear of venereal infection may alter libido:

(1)   Where the lady partner has been infected by a sexual relationship of her own making - regular or casual partner - and required treatment.

(2)   Where the woman has a phobia for infections in general, and genital infections in particular, so-called venerophobia.

(3)   Where the patient suffers from obsessive-compulsive disorder, in which hygiene rituals are part of the symptomatology.

(4)   An occasional example is the young (or older) sexually in-experienced woman, who has developed some symptoms soon after coitus but does not discuss these with her family doctor or indeed with her sexual partner. She simply lets her sexual interest and drive wane as a self-protective mechanism. Thus an innocent leukorrhoea, or a transient itch, may proceed to libidinal suppres-sion and loss of sexual outlet.

(5)   Where the woman discovers her male partner has, or carries, AIDS virus.

PERFORMANCE ANXIETIES

Performance anxiety may refer to the woman's own performance, or to her anticipation of the male partner's performance, or both. The rising expectations in sexual relationships for pleasure, fun, happiness, even ecstacy, as well as the anticipation of orgasm in the woman and ejaculation in the male partner, may mean that neither partner will settle for limited return in the sexual setting. Disappointment with her own response may arise in the following patterns:

Failure to relax and lubricate easily.

Failure to enjoy intromission and the sense of coupling as a unit.

Failure to desire to respond to the verbal and action endearments of the partner in the coital process.

Failure to reach 'a point of no return' with sheer sensual delight and a feeling of floating away with joy.

Failure to experience orgasmic contractions within and of the genital tract.

Failure to look forward to the next sexual encounter.

The woman may also experience a let down in her partner's performance such as:

Absence of stimulating foreplay.

Failure to consider pleasure of erotic areas or best coital positioning.

Too rapid intromission.

Too rapid ejaculation.

Failure to stay awake and enjoy the after-glow of sex.

Interruption of the sex act by his donning a condom.

Request for deviational acts - anal sex, cross dressing, for example.

Bad choice of environment.

Excessive intake of alcohol prior to coitus.

Inability to achieve erection or maintain full erection.

Absence of ejaculate.

Accepting that sex is not invariably a wonderful experience, performance anxiety may derive from a genuine unwillingness to make love on her partner's side, disturbed ability to enjoy and concentrate on sensations, and an inability to relax. The latter is followed by a sense of watchfulness derived from bad memories of the previous sexual encounter. This moves on to the total absence of spontaneity and is replaced by anxiety at each stage of coitus. Another component of this problem which can affect libido is that of anger - one partner blames the other for poor performance and poor satisfaction. Efforts at discussion become minimal, and sexual communication may come to a standstill. A sense of hopelessness may further depress libido. Some women in this situation become vulnerable to the approach of sympathetic listeners of the opposite sex and are tempted away from the regular partnership, likewise the male partner.

Performance anxiety may also be a part of another source of libido suppression or depression, fear of discovery. Privacy for sexual intercourse permits an easy, relaxed and leisurely enjoyment of foreplay and coitus. Absence of privacy, for many couples, places a strain on the form and content of the sexual encounter. If this is ongoing, then the woman may find, her partner too, that the libido is altered in a negative direction. Examples of lack of privacy include:

Premarital couple invariably chaperoned by parents or relatives.

Premarital couple using 'borrowed' premises, car or caravan.

Premarital couple on holiday with their families.

Married couple with children who 'wander in' the bedroom or won't settle to sleep.

Married couple with parents and in-laws, who stay with them (or vice versa).

Older married couple living with married child.

Older married couple in residential care.

Extramarital meetings in any situation.

COSMETIC TURN-OFFS

The balance between what turns on a woman's sexuality and drive and what turns it off, in relation to her partner, can be a fine one. Whereas a woman's nudity or partial nudity has long been considered to elevate sexual desire in the male observer, male nudity may or may not be exciting for the female observer. The cosmetic view of her male partner may be stimulating in libido terms - examples include the 'trouser bulge', the swimsuit trunks, the hairy or hairless chest, general muscularity, hair style or scalp hair nudity. The penis size, length, firmness and presence or absence of foreskin may all be positive reinforcers of sexual tension in the lady partner.

Cosmetic turn-offs may be thought of as 'obvious' - gross obesity, 'pot belly', short stature, baldness, grey hair, motor handicap, bad breath, dental caries, for example. They may be more 'subtle' - manner of speech, use of perfumes, wearing a beard, pipe smoking, poor hygiene of nails and body, for example. Cosmetic changes are a feature of ageing, and the lady partner may dislike what advancing chronology does to her male lover: wrinkling, sagging, stooping, slowing, loss of teeth, need to wear specs or hearing aid, use of walking aid, for example. Ablative surgery may exacerbate these assorted feelings and depress the libido. Colostomy and ileostomy, amputation of digits or limbs, abdominal or chest scars from operations, herniotomy and orchidectomy are typical examples which provoke an attitude of 'turn off'. The problem may be compounded by awareness of her own ageing changes in similar cosmetic terms. She may feel that her partner could no longer fancy her at all, become depressed at this unspoken thought, and down goes the libido.

Illness in the woman herself may be a turn-off. This may be in the short-term of an acute illness or in the longer term of a chronic illness. It is not, however, invariable for all women. Sometimes a particular illness focuses the woman's eyes on what is, and what is not, pleasing and pleasurable. She may feel that sex gives her some compensation for the health disturbance. As we have already discussed under the male problems heading, fear of exacerbating an illness or of causing it to recur may also depress loving feelings and sexual drive. The woman may also be turned off by the presence of a disease process in her partner. This can be true whether or not such a disease or complaint produces visible external changes in the man, like weight loss, pallor, muscle weakness, or not.

That mental illness can alter libido, we have already considered and discussed under the same heading in the male partner section of this book. The illnesses that can alter libido include anxiety states, neuroses, mania and depression as well as schizophrenia and organic dementia. The alteration is generally in a negative direction but we have also described the (less common) hypersexuality states that can ensue. Dementing disinhibited women can, like their male counterparts, expose themselves or masturbate or behave sexually in an inappropriate antisocial way. This is unpleasant but, strangely, appears to distress families and carers less than if the same behaviour is undertaken in the male subject.

Aversion has also been fully considered earlier, as some researchers view it, in male and female terms. The primary and secondary forms appear in women as well as in men. Libido can be restored as the aversion is treated.

RELIGION

The significance of religion in relation to sexual drive, sexual tension and outlet is liable to be overlooked or played down in Western society because secular influences have apparently become so dominant.

Nevertheless, there remain large groups of society whose practice and precepts lean heavily on religious or religio-ethnic views of what is proper and acceptable, in premarriage and within marriage. These codes of behaviour are passed on from one generation to the next, fortified by the leaders of the religious movement - minister or priest, for example. In some religions, sex and sexuality are considered valuable and relevant parts of life within a family setting. In other religions, sex is permissible for procreation or potential conception but viewed as linked with sin, corruption, evil or potential wickedness if being undertaken purely for pleasure. The separation of sex and love is in practice a difficult one for many religions.

The girl or woman who is brought up in a strongly religious setting, and who fails to match her partner to this type of background and practice, may run into moral and practical difficulties in her sex life. More so is this a feature, when she herself decides to 'break away' from her religious upbringing and customs and make her own choices in this and other areas of life. Under some circumstances of sexual encounter and activity a sense of guilt may be engendered. This religious guilt can, in some women, act to reduce a previously satisfactory libido. It represents another form of anxiety state in that respect and may ultimately be resolved by several approaches to anxiety effect on libido that we shall consider later.

PREGNANCY – AGAIN

Three decades ago, the traditional teaching to medical students and the consequent advice by qualified doctors, recommended against sexual intercourse for the pregnant woman in the first and in the third trimester. Later views suggested that, unless the partner had an infection, or unless the pregnant woman had placenta praevia or other potentially serious intrauterine or health problems, coitus (including orgasm) could proceed right up to term with no likely ill effects. These medical attitudes did not necessarily, if at all, match with the regular practices or attitudes of the pregnant woman within her partnership.

Contemporary studies about activity or anxieties in pregnancy related to sexuality seem to indicate that one woman in four has no great change in her sex life during pregnancy. (We are not here talking about the mechanics of coitus that may require positional adjustment.) About 50% of women do report a reduction in frequency of sexual activity and coitus. The libido can alter in pregnancy, however, but the reports suggest the figure for those with lowered libido is one in every 14 expectant mothers. For some of this group, and indeed some of the reduced coitus group, the pattern derives from fear of health risk to mother and baby, or some degree of guilt at enjoying sexuality in her pregnant state. In relation to our look at religious influence on libido, the studies of coital frequency in pregnancy failed to show any association with racial, religious or ethnic groups.

As a counter to the likelihood of libido suppression, the original Masters and Johnson study of female sexuality in pregnancy, reported in the 1960s, suggested an increase in sexual desire and outlet during the second trimester in a high percentage of women. Subsequent researchers reduced this 'high' figure to about 25%.

MENOPAUSE AND PMT

Menopausal 'upset' is a common midlife problem and yet many women decline to seek help or advice from the family doctor, believing that he will view her complaints as silly, neurotic, or untreatable in any case. Appearing at a women's reproductive life anywhere between her late thirties and her early fifties, the symptoms of the menopause may be mild, moderate or marked, short-term or prolonged. The accepted features, indicating the run-down of ovarian function and depletion of female sex hormone, include hot flushes day or night, dryness or irritation of the vagina, muscle aches and muscle weakness, headache, ligament laxity. To these can be added neurotic upset, psychosomatic upset and psychotic illness.

The woman whose emotional state has long been maladjusted can certainly produce neurotic symptoms at the menopause. Complaints of feeling anxious, tense, unable to sleep, palpitation, giddiness, pins and needles may appear, plus a general malaise that persists from one 'Monday morning' to the next. Careful questioning and gentle enquiry may reveal a whole series of fears: no more an ability to mother as well as conceive; no longer sexually in bloom and attractive; no stopping the ageing process; no guarantees against loneliness if her husband rejects her; no making up for lost possibilities in sexual and loving terms, are typical examples.

The adjusted and stable woman is only modestly affected, if at all, by the departure of ovarian function. Freed from monthly periods, freed from the chances of pregnancy, freed from household ties, she may turn her freedom into energetic outgoing pursuits of either paid or voluntary activities. Instead of putting her partner off by a catalogue of woes, she can encourage him and support him in new directions. Whereas the libido of the emotionally maladjusted woman may nosedive, the libido of this stable lady remains firm and may lift further.

Psychiatrists who have closely studied the menopausal syndrome invariably advise us not to assume that all somatic symptoms are simply 'the change'. Many physical diseases appear or are exacerbated in middle years, such as diabetes, the thyroid disorders, hypertension, and the anaemias. The patient with loss of libido at the menopause may therefore have an organic disorder, unrelated to oestrogen deficiency. This implies that we must give a full clinical assessment to the woman before pronouncing on the menopause as source.

True psychosis can appear for the first time at the menopause or represent a resurgence of earlier mental disorder. Depression is the most familiar of the severe illnesses of mental life that occur as a slow insidious disturbance. Late schizophrenia and paranoia can also occur at this life period. These in turn may affect libido, as we have noted before.

Another 'hormonal' syndrome, nowadays regarded with more care and seriousness than 20 years ago, is that of premenstrual tension. Three out of four women regularly and predictably experience one or more symptomatic upsets in the 12-14 days prior to the onset of menstruation. This PMT, as it is labelled, can include autonomic upsets like nausea, sickness, sweating, flushing and feeling giddy or faint. It can include fluid retention with bloated stomach, puffy painful breasts and weight gain. It may include myalgic and arthritic features affecting neck and back, as well as headache, irritability and weeping spells. Problems of concentration and insomnia may appear. We might view reasonably that this collection of emotional and somatic features would invariably depress libido. This is possible and realistic. Yet other women show no change in libido, or even manifest an increase in desire and activity as if to enjoy life to the full before the newest menstruation spoils it all.

VAGINISMUS

In sexuality, among the oldest recognized female disturbances of psychosomatic origin, vaginismus is named. This has long been separated from other forms of painful or allegedly painful intercourse because of its five characteristics:

(1) When vaginal penetration by the penis is attempted, involuntary contraction in spasm takes place in the vaginal muscles.

(2) The muscles which contract are those of the perineum and outer third of the vagina.

(3) The sufferer opts for external sanitary protection at menstruation and avoids tampons, that is, internal sanitary protection.

(4) The sufferer invariably avoids self-exploration or examination of her vulvovaginal area.

(5) Internal examination by the gynaecologist or family doctor is usually avoided or, if insisted upon, invariably unsatisfactory.

Vaginismus usually appears in the early weeks or months of a first relationship for the woman. The woman may initially be aroused and even be climaxed by her partner as part of manual or oral petting, but as soon as first penetration by the penis is undertaken, however gently and thoughtfully by the male partner, involuntary vaginal muscle spasm places a 'no entry' sign up. As time goes on, further efforts by the partner simply reinforce the vaginismus response, and non-consummation is the order of the day. Of course, pregnancy and conception may ensue without full penetration. In that case, the vaginismus may come to light on vaginal examination attempts at the antenatal clinic. Neither does labour and delivery guarantee a cure of the vaginismus, which can readily recur in the first new coitus after the baby's first few weeks. We shall look at therapy later but the persistence of vaginismus may alter the libido of both partners, not just the woman who experiences it.

ORGANIC DISCOMFORTS

The five criteria of vaginismus notwithstanding, it is important to exclude other elements which might cause uncomfortable coitus. These may be organic, such as we shall now consider, or may be emotional in terms of marital discord, anxiety neurosis or depression. The initial interview gives an opportunity to take a clinical as well as sexual history, if not yet known, and assess clinically other body systems as well as the genital system.

Organic agencies which may depress or suppress libido run parallel to those that we have seen in the male partner. Local genital infection in women, which may affect sexual drive and sexual interest, may appear *de novo*, or have been transmitted in sexual relationships with one or more partners. They include the following:

Non-specific urethritis and vulvovaginitis (most often chlamydia)
Gonococcal infection of urethra and genital tract
Syphilitic infection of the genital tract

Vaginal candida (thrush)
Vaginal trichomonas
Genital warts
Pubic lice
Molluscum contagiosum
Chancroid, lymphogranuloma venereum, granuloma inguinale - all rarer.

Local and systemic therapy may be required, and the reader is referred to an appropriate book on sexually transmitted illness for further details. When treatment is successful but the libido fails to return, then further counselling is clearly indicated. Local scarring causing pain, and anxiety or mild depression, may derive from episiotomy scars, local herniotomy scars, prolapse or other operative scars. A referral to the original surgeon may be valuable whether to gynaecologist or general surgeon. The presence of scars does not invariably confirm organic pain.

DRUGS – AGAIN

The effects of drugs and the side-effects of drugs are most readily seen in male sexuality with secondary problems of erection and ejaculation. Centrally acting drugs such as tranquillizers, hypnotics and antidepressants may - in their action of calming, relieving insomnia and reversing gloom and apathy - happily alter the libido in a positive direction. Alternatively, they may reduce the capacity and speed of arousal in some women and so fail to promote libido at all. Antidepressants were seen in the male subject to interfere with ejaculation but parallel negative reports against effective orgasm are not readily forthcoming in female subjects.

Women suffering from epilepsy can, like their male counterparts, lose libidinal drive as a consequence of taking anticonvulsants. Those who take clonidine, for menopausal flushing or for hypertension, may risk mild depression and consequently altered libido. The same goes for the use of methyldopa in hypertension. Those who use cimetidine for peptic oesophagitis or for alimentary peptic ulcer are unlikely to have depressed libido, since there is some evidence of a raised serum testosterone. Women suffering from undue hirsutism and placed on cyproterone can have an altered libido, thanks to its antiandrogen effect.

Disturbed arousal and orgasmic disturbance are theoretically possible in the use of digitalis and diuretics, but are not usually so reported by patients. The use of hormone replacement therapy at the menopause certainly improves the local genital tract and may increase a feeling of well-being. Depressed libido may still require the short-term addition of androgens, however, the sequential oestrogens and progestogens notwithstanding. As with psychologically induced erectile dysfunction in men, so women with altered libido or anorgasmia may blame the medication for the problem as a handy excuse - an excuse that proves not to be borne out on closer study.

ALCOHOL

The influence of alcohol on sexual drive and sexual capacity has already been considered in the male partner. Its dual capacity to disinhibit the individual and permit greater arousal while sometimes centrally lowering functional capacity are more noticeable in men. The effects are parallel in women so that greater receptivity and ease of coital interaction may be noted in some woman partakers of alcohol but the response in an orgasmic sense may be lessened or even absent.

Excessive and heavy drinking is known to induce earlier changes of cirrhosis and risk of liver failure than in men. This potential can be translated into chronic illhealth, which in turn recognizably reduces or causes loss of libido. The association of alcoholism with depression is no less likely in some women than in some men, especially if there is a past history of affective disorder. Here again, the libido will suffer as the woman becomes apathetic, withdrawn, disinterested and self-neglectful.

We have also noted that peripheral neuropathy can be the end result of excessive alcohol intake, especially if associated with poor diet and lack of vitamin B intake. It is not clear whether, in women, such neuropathic changes influence functional activity in a direct sense. Indirectly it represents another source of disease which may suppress libidinal interest.

We have also considered how alcohol users may turn to illegal drugs usage as part of, or alternative to, a particular life style. The same factors regarding such drugs and their effect on sexuality as we noted in men are paralleled in women users. In contemporary times, the teenage and adult user of illicit drugs is just as likely to be a woman as a man. In some partnerships, there is joint abuse of alcohol or joint abuse of illegal drugs - or both.

THE PILL

The hormonal contraceptive pill, although not being used for any organic disease or disability, is still in the medical sense a drug. The 1974 survey in the United Kingdom by family doctors suggested that women using the oral hormonal contraceptive approach were nearly four times more likely to report sexual problems than the women who used other birth control methods. This view of a possible adverse effect on libido, or other elements in female sexuality, did not match earlier studies which suggested higher levels of sexual activity in contraceptive 'pill users'. Subsequent workers have suggested that, while subtle responses and changes in hormonal status may affect individuals, there is no universal upset of sexual desire and arousal in all women having oral contraception.

PHYSICAL ILLNESSES

Physical illhealth, as we have already seen in the male partner, can produce a short-term or more prolonged depression of libido and sexual capacity and outlet. This means that all doctors invariably meet sexual problems in their daily practice, although sometimes patients fail to voice their difficulties or report the changes until almost too late or too painful. In a given disease, discomfort or pain, weakness or fatigue, poor mobility or immobility, anxiety over outcome and depression at the presence of the illness may all, or in any combination, reduce sexual interest and sexual drive. For some women whose libido is already low or whose pleasure from sexual activity is minimal, illness may be a reasonable excuse to bring such activity to an end and keep the partner at bay. In other cases, the recovery from physical illness may see a natural return of libido and the couple simply taking up sexually where they had left off.

Altered appearance from physical illness may affect self-esteem and confidence and create fear of rejection. Examples include skin complaints of face and trunk, scars, ablative surgery - ostomies - and pigmentary changes.

CHRONIC DISEASES

When we review the various body system illnesses of a more chronic variety, we can recognize a number of significant points in relation to libido change.

In chronic obstructive airway disease, the decreasing respiration efficiency can result in dyspnoea in the arousal, plateau or orgasm phases of coitus. This may be off-putting. Where coitus is usually undertaken in the horizontal position, lung expansion and mucus collection problems can also mechanically disturb the coital progress. In bronchial asthma of any severity, the excitement of coitus can be an inducing factor for an attack, as with any other form of vigorous exercise.

In chronic renal failure with uraemia, the patient treated on dialysis may, as we have noted in the male partner section, feel physically improved but fail to show a rise in libido or in sexual arousal capacity. Excessive prolactin in such patients can be antiandrogenic which again may lower the libido of the woman with renal desease. Consideration of bromocriptine therapy to counter the high prolactin levels may reverse the libido's downwards trend.

The same problem of excessive prolactin turns up in cirrhotic illness of the liver with secondary hepatic failure. Libido falls and output diminishes. Associated absence of menstrual periods or scanty menstruation is not uncommon. In some of these women, an additional factor is that the cirrhosis is due to chronic alcoholism, itself a potent cause of disturbed sexual drive and sexual function. Ischaemic heart disease particularly with angina may reduce libido by the tiredness and fatigue effect, or by pain in the chest coming on with arousal, or with coital activity. The feeling of dyspnoea and palpitation in cardiac patients during intercourse may act to lower libidinal interest.

Clearly then, physical illhealth can affect the libido through its alteration of the affect, as well as through direct effect on one or more of the controlling physiological mechanisms. We have seen how, in the male partner, diabetes mellitus can have multiple contributing factors in disturbing sexual function and sexual drive. Whereas such upsets may begin to affect male diabetics within 5-6 years of having the illnesss, sexual dysfunction in women takes between 6 and 10 years to reveal itself. One diabetic woman in three is less likely to complain or report that orgasm is less frequent, or has become absent altogether. As a consequence, and especially if the diabetic woman herself links this change to her illness, the libido may become depressed.

In the undiagnosed diabetic woman or in the unstable diabetic woman, there may be loss of sexual drive or dissatisfaction with sexual feelings in coitus. The correction or treatment of diabetes mellitus may restore the situation to the previous level of libido. Diabetic women are more subject to intertrigo, groin and perivulval infections, often with thrush. This can mechanically affect the comfort of coitus. As always it should not be overlooked that diabetics, like other men and women, can experience emotional and psychological sexual dysfunction without hard evidence of diabetic organic effects.

Urinary tract infections, as we have seen already in terms of urethritis and cystitis, can, from first 'honeymoon' coitus, create sexual upset and affect libido. There may be anatomical and physiological as well as pathological local factors, encouraging dyspareunia which need expert attention.

Osteoarthritis and rheumatoid arthritis can give pain and coital discomfort and thereby reduce libido. Symptomatic and idiopathic epileptic fits can create loss of libido even before any drug side-effects may do so. Degenerative central nervous system illness like multiple sclerosis can do likewise.

Apart from diabetes mellitus, other endocrinopathies can affect sexual desire and sexual outlet. Thyroxine is necessary for the metabolic function of all body cells, and hypothyroidism includes in its effects not just cardiac and alimentary features of bodily slowing down by also amenorrhoea and loss of sexual desire and drive. Theoretically, thyrotoxicosis might be associated with increased libido since there is an upsurge of general metabolic activity. Most probably, the associated autonomic disturbance puts paid to any thyroxine excess 'aphrodisiac' effect, and the libido still ends up on the reduced or absent scale.

Hypogonadal changes from Simmond's disease, or panhypo-pituitarism, are accompanied by loss of the menses and infertility. These alone may not necessarily dampen libido. The associated lack of thyroid stimulating hormone and adrenocorticotrophic hormone cumu-latively invite a loss of sexual stimulation and interest. Paradoxically, in this infertile state, some women show an increased interest in becoming pregnant which is oddly divorced from the state of the sexual drive. In primary Addison's disease, or hypoadrenalism, the libido is particularly likely to be depressed since the woman relies on this set of glands as a rich source of androgens. It is usual to point out that standard steroid substitution therapy in primary hypoadrenal states will not effectively lift the libido. Additional androgen replacement may be required.

SURGERY EFFECTS

Surgical therapy of illness such as cervical ulcer and uterine polyps, removal of local carcinomas, hysterectomy, and treatment of prolapse may all be followed by temporary loss of libido. Unless there is local pain or discomfort, or loss of mobility or inability to have deep penetration, coitus should be possible when libido returns. The psychological effects of surgery - anxiety, fear, ideas of cosmetic turn-off, ideas of loss of feminity - may conspire to hold down or remove sexual desire and interest.

Understanding Sexual Medicine

We have already looked at the psychological and emotional effects of the menopause. The physical changes vary according to the degree of drop in oestrogen levels. Vulval atrophy with thinned pubic hair is accompanied by drying of the vaginal walls and poor lubricatory responses in the sexual situation. There is increased vulnerability to local infection which can add to pain or discomfort in coitus. The cosmetic change may also be upsetting for the woman, whose sexual orientation towards her own body is linked with a particular image that she understands as attractive to the male partner.

The postnatal state of womanhood can apparently affect the libido in a variety of ways which may be 'classified' as both psychological or organic. The return of libido (or the eagerness of the male partner) may be expressed by questions to the family doctor on how soon intercourse can be resumed. While a figure of 6 weeks postpartum is often mentioned, many couples make their own decision. Women who choose to breast-feed their babies might be thought, on first consideration, to have a lowered interest in coitus, in view of the concentration on the baby's needs, the presence of 'wet' breasts, and the mechanics of coitus which avoid 'wet' breast handling. There seems to be no clear difference between postnatal women who breast-feed and bottle-feed, however, in the degree of sexual interest expressed. Studies conflict in this area, some suggesting no great alteration with breast feeding, others even suggesting a greater return of libido in breast-feeders.

In some postnatal women, the appearance of 'puerperal' depression may depress the libido. The depression requires urgent therapy. In some postnatal women, fear of further pregnancy too soon after this one may keep sexual interest and drive to low levels. This can be true whether the pregnancy was uneventful or not. The fatigue of her care of the neonate may also lower sexual drive.

6
Disability, Handicap and Sexuality

HANDICAP AND DISABILITY

In preceding chapters, we have taken a broad and sometimes specific look at acquired disability, from disease processes or drugs or psychological disturbances. In this chapter, we can consider the boys and girls, or men and women of the adult community, who have been born with motor or sensory handicaps, or disabilities of communication, or varying degrees of intellectual retardation. The traditional and sometimes persisting view of sexuality, in congenital or birth-injured citizens, is one of absent sexual drive, low sexual interest and absent sexual outlet. They are - to quote George Lee - merely seen as contented invalids with only spiritual interests. Such a view, until very recent years, led to a conspiracy of silence over any sexual problems or expressed sexual needs, whether the handicapped citizen was kept at home or was mobile in a limited way, or lived in residential homes or in hospital care settings. This suppression of information, or anxieties or experience of sexual frustration, was exacerbated in citizens who were unable to relocate from a wheelchair or a bed.

Even when sexual outlet was clearly required, the chances of a disabled man or woman undertaking love-making were made more remote by the following:

(1)   Absence of a suitable social setting showing sufficient privacy.
(2)   The nature of the disability in relation to full coitus.
(3)   The problem of overcoming social rejection.

The last comes about because of society's blinkered and unrealistic view, that the most suitable or even perfect partner has an attractive body, a sound mind and full physical integrity. Never mind the partners themselves who may love and enjoy each other's company and views, and share physical pleasures. Never mind the disabled person's view that reaching out to the non-disabled is likely to be rebuffed.

We may even add that the possible infertility, or undesirability of pregnancy and parenthood in certain forms of handicap has been a source, tacitly or covertly agreed to indicate non-sexuality - in motor, sensory or mentally handicapped citizens of both sexes.

If that is the picture adopted by able-bodied citizens, we can hardly be surprised that many disabled youngsters themselves have failed to seek counsel or aid, or support or information in areas of sexuality. Family doctors and hospital doctors who come regularly, or periodically, in contact with disabled and handicapped youngsters (and oldsters) have only recently been prepared to take serious and positive interest in sexual function and sexual dysfunction of this far from homogeneous population group.

TYPE OF PROBLEMS

In the United Kingdom, the work of the organization called SPOD (sexual problems of the disabled and elderly), the research and support lent by the Spastics Society and Spina Bifida Society, and the interest of many voluntary groups like the Multiple Sclerosis Society and the Ileostomy Association, have collectively helped to develop and sustain progress in this area of human sexuality. Departments of physical medicine and rehabilitation, units caring for paraplegics and tetraplegics, departments caring for infertility and sterility, have likewise been involved in the practical aspects of sexual communication, sexual contact, coitus, psychosocial problems and partnership difficulties. The breadth of such problems may range from teaching arousal and penis 'capture' techniques to the non-handicapped female partner of a male paraplegic, to gauging the best position for physical contact by two spastic partners, to controlling micturition in a spinal cord injury patient who wishes to continue full coitus, and on to the correction of social isolation or poor sexual self-image in motor or other handicapped young people.

The range of handicaps is so wide that the associative sexual difficulties are not readily classified into a few straightforward categories. For example, the congenitally blind boy or girl has to learn about the anatomical differences of male and female in an alternative approach to straight picturing and visual identification. The arousal stage is stimulated not by the sight of nudity, near-nudity, provocative clothing or erotic movements but by touch, odour, speech and various sounds. Coital contact can be guided by a sighted partner but has to be more skilfully learned and guided if both partners are unsighted.

Or, for example, the congenitally deaf young man or woman cannot pick up the sexual signals and sexual responses of a verbal or sound nature which appear in those of normal hearing. They can see and appreciate visual expressions of eroticism in a general sense. Their isolation in adolescent development may prevent the usual internalizing of the normal taboos related to sexuality. Differences of hearing in a hearing handicapped couple can lead to misunderstandings, jealousy or discord in relation to sexual communication before, during or after the sexual act.

Or, for example, the congenitally spastic man or woman who chooses to partner a similarly motor handicapped citizen, may find that incoordination and adductor muscle spasm preclude or frustrate efforts at sexual intercourse. Counselling may then involve conjoint discussion of alternative expressions of loving contact of breasts and genitals - oral sex in its varied forms. It might include forms of mutual masturbation. It may also consider the use of mechanical aids.

In the three foregoing examples, we talk of partners but sexual advice may be sought by the unattached or lone handicapped citizen as well.

Such an individual may have locomotor problems, motor difficulties, balance upset, face or limb or trunk abnormalities, slower mentality, for

(1)   example, and be looking for aid in five areas:

(2)   Understanding their own degree of sexual feelings.

(3)   Finding an acceptable and available form of sexual outlet.

(4)   Understanding how the opposite sex views sexuality.

        Reassurance regarding health, infection risks, pregnancy risks, social acceptability, of any partnered sexual activities which may
(5)   become available.

        Seeking the doctor's support against any parental or institutional resistance to sociosexual partnering.

Looked at in broad terms, the differences between the congenital handicap and the acquired disability resemble the differences between primary and secondary sexual dysfunction - the former starting with a vacuum which may or may not be filled, the latter having known something or a great deal of experience and activity but now having to adjust (alone or in partnership) to the specific changes imposed by the handicap.

AN APPROACH

In many countries, the specialized services required for neurological handicap, congenital and acquired, were forced to recognize sexual issues. Whether they adopt one-to-one interviews or group sessions, the same questions are presented to the experts. Examples include:

> Is it fair to the partner to continue the relationship with a handicapped man or woman?

> Is it possible to have sexual feelings and desires yet have no erectile or orgasmic functional capacity?

> How do I cope with my absence of sexual experience till now?

> How can I go on expressing my need and love for my partner?

> How can I be sure my partner is still happy/satisfied sexually?

These questions can be equally applicable in many other forms of handicap or disabling illness.

The family doctor whose aid is sought in this field of sexuality can bring his combination of medical and psychosocial skills into good use. His awareness of the individual setting of the family, their health and welfare history, their cultural background, and their likely intellectual levels, permits him to judge what can be done at primary care level with his team and what requires referral to other experts - psychologist, psychiatrist, other sexual counsellor, marriage guidance counsellor, for example. Even after referral to other experts, the follow through of the efforts of such individuals will inevitably require monitoring and supporting by a good primary care team.

Of interest in relationship to the whole topic of sex and disability, is the fact that the organizations dealing with such handicaps have - like SPOD - come to include sexuality of the older citizen. This is because the onset of later life brings degeneration of various systems - locomotor, respiratory, cardiac, endocrine, genital - and decline of muscular vigour, as well as altered social roles, and increasing loss of partners. Reduced acceptance by society at large of any expression of libido and sexual activity in an old man or woman creates further difficulties.

Whatever the nature of the congenital handicap, five factors are required to achieve a successful sexual relationship:

(1)   The presence of mutually willing partners, disabled or not.

(2)   A place of privacy to meet - with suitable environmental con-

ditions to satisfy the mental and physical aspects of the relationship.

(3)   Ability to discuss openly difficulties arising between themselves.

(4)   Opportunity and willingness to try various alternative patterns of sexual contact or expression.

(5)   Available expert counselling, with or without actual human on-the-spot aid.

7
Therapies and Counselling

THERAPEUTIC APPROACHES TO SEXUAL DYSFUNCTION

En route, in our consideration of the anatomy and physiology and psychology of sex as well as the common sexual problems in men and women, we have sometimes noted therapies and forseen the possibilities for correction, control or cure of dysfunctions. There has been evidence also that some complaints are likely to be irreversible while others only may require shorter or more prolonged and time-consuming attention to influence the outcome in a positive direction. In this chapter we can now take a general and more specific look at the following therapy aspects:

Where and how do the problems present in family practice?

Where and how can the family doctor offer help, advice and counsel?

What special questions do we need to ask in beginning our counselling?

Are there fixed approaches to some problems?

Should some patients be referred to other experts, and if so, to whom?

What criteria of success can we use?

Studies in general practice and the individual experience of GPs, suggest that relatively few patients come directly to ask for help in sexual areas. (Those who indirectly ask for help do so in the guise of therapy for somatic complaints, or advice on contraception, advice on child management, enquiries about drug therapy, for example.) One reason given for this small number of direct queries is that many couples will ignore the quality and satisfaction - or lack of it - in a sexual relationship until there is a major life change, or a significant social change, or a very specific sexual dysfunction appears that can be pinpointed, such as loss of erection or severe dyspareunia. When the latter takes place, either or both partners may finally communicate sufficiently to decide on a policy of aid, and thereafter visit the family doctor.

It has been suggested that more sexual problems or difficulties in sexual relationships would be uncovered if a few questions on sex were asked routinely in history taking for any clinical problem. This would, in theory, offer the patient a direct lead - even if it was apparently digressing from the main problem - into the arena of sexuality. Routine enquiries about sexuality are not included in the clinical training of medical undergraduates, except in obvious areas like genitourinary medicine, contraception or menstrual dysfunction, for example. Most doctors would not therefore regard any questions on sexual function as 'legitimate' in routine clinical problems. Oppositely, it has been the case that patients would open up the matter of sexual dysfunction with family doctors, or even hospital 'non-sex problems' specialists, only to be thwarted by that doctor side-stepping or re-channelling the discussion away from sexual matters.

The family doctor who has taken instruction or attended lectures in sexual problems, as well as those naturally at ease with the topic, can register the direct or indirect query on sexuality. He can then decide whether to utilize the available surgery time left for that patient and extend the topic to see where it leads. Alternatively, he can ask the patient to re-attend surgery at the end of the appointments schedule on a given day, to permit a longer interview session. Family doctors with a special interest in sex counselling may hold a special surgery session for this purpose, assuming there are sufficient patients who would utilize this extra-clinical endeavour. No special label need be placed on this clinic. It could also be run in parallel with family planning or antenatal sessions, if considered appropriate. Advantages of the latter presumably lie in seeing partners rather than individuals - if that is what the patient desires.

PATTERNS OF PRESENTING PROBLEMS

Whether the patient comes to ask for direct help, or gives an 'oh by the way, can I ask you about...' enquiry at the end of the appointment time, or whether the patient leaves his or her innuendo to 'let the penny drop' for you - there appear to be four patterns in the problems so presented.

The first pattern is a report of a specific loss of sexual capacity or altered sexual capacity. Examples include absence of erection, inability to hold an erection, loss of lubrication, or deep dyspareunia. The second pattern is a report of partner incompatibility in the sexual needs, sexual performance and sexual outlet of the man and woman. The third pattern is a report of loss of libido or of sexual aversion or both. The last pattern is a report of intramarital discord and difficulties, in which sexual disturbance is only one of several discordant areas.

If the last pattern quickly becomes apparent, the doctor may have to decide whether he should refer the couple to a marriage guidance counsellor and invite them back once the partnership is more stable. Alternatively, he may consider that the sexual problem can be fairly quickly corrected - for example, premature ejaculation or drug-induced anorgasmia - and then he will refer the couple on to the marriage guidance area. It is also possible but not easy, to run the sexual counselling in parallel with the couple's attendance at the marriage guidance sessions.

Family doctors may have found that a discordant couple will, as in the marriage guidance setting, seek to use him as judge and jury on the guilt of one or other partner, in relation to the sexual disturbance sector of their disharmony. Finding a middle unprejudiced way in such a situation may not be easy, but can be significant in a therapeutic sense. The same call for 'guilty' judgement arises in the sexual incompatibility pattern, mentioned secondly above.

HISTORY TAKING

In clinical diagnosis in general medicine, we usually ask the patient to tell us ' the problem' or the complaint in his or her own words. We are taught not to lead the patient or put ideas into his mouth. Medical skill permits us to modify that strict ruling in many circumstances, most obviously with older citizens, those of lower intellect and those whose illness produces problems of communication. In sexual medicine, we again ask the patient to present the problem in his or her own words. No matter how intellectually bright, mentally clear, youthful or old the patient may be, offering a report on intimate sexual difficulties is rarely straightforward for the patient. Lack of specific vocabulary, fear of embarrassing the doctor by using jargon or street argot in sexual terms, difficulty in emphasizing what is going wrong because of ignorance of genital anatomy, are all elements that may force the doctor to take a lead in the process of finding out the details of the problem. The ability of the doctor to defuse the emotion of the situation, to make the patient feel at ease, to convince the patient of the confidential nature of this interview, can make the difference between most of the sexual truth being revealed or merely the tip of the sexual iceberg.

Where little progress in history taking is being made, or where there is stumbling and stuttering over the material to be presented, a useful ploy is to reassure the man or woman that you are going to help them even if they find it hard or awkward to talk. You are going to make it easier by asking 'ten simple questions' to which they only need say 'yes' or 'no'. This short questionnaire should, by these positive or negative replies, permit you to move towards a rounded view of the complaint, and on to the appropriate clinical and sexual examination that is required.

Here are the ten questions, for a 'yes' or 'no':

(1)   Has the problem only appeared within the last 4 weeks?

(2)   Is the problem present on every sexual occasion?

(3)   Has your general health been good?

(4)   Are you taking any doctor-prescribed or self-prescribed drugs?

(5)   Is there one sexual partner only?

(6)   Have you sought advice from other sources?

(7)   Have you come to see me on your own initiative?

(8)   Have you had any sex instruction in any form?

(9)   Have you strong sexual feelings?

(10) Are you prepared to spend regular time each week for therapy?

This group of questions is structured to find a balance between the attending patient's genuine wish to be helped or not, and confirmation of some key elements in sexual disturbance like organic illness, drugs, lack of knowledge, and lack of sexual drive.

Combining the patient's own history with the simple questionnaire, the counselling doctor can write down a provisional assessment of the problem, not just as a single label of, say, erection upset or absent orgasm but as a descriptive picture. Here are three examples:

Menopausal 48 year old, one partner, reduced libido, lubrication loss.

Remarried recently, 31 year old man, modest libido, premature ejaculation.

42 year old colitis man, with recent ileostomy, anxious, poor erection, marital and extramarital partners.

Such a descriptive approach keeps us in mind of the patient as a whole, rather than using a purely medical model of disease labelling and ignoring the strongly linked psychosocial aspects. Where the partner has come along, the doctor may make a general assessment of her role, attitudes, experience, drive and love for her affected partner in the case of the male subject - and vice versa. Keeping the unaffected partner informed of your counselling intentions as well as the patient can be valuable in any treatment regime.

THE CLINICAL EXAMINATION

Whether the patient presents alone or with the partner, a full clinical examination, following the opening interview to assess history and problem, is undertaken. This is a major advantage that the medical sex counsellor enjoys over non-medical counsellors. It permits an opportunity to assess physical sexual maturity, the presence or absence of possible contributing organic factor, the patient's attitude to his or her own body and especially to his or her genitalia, and reassurance on the normality of organ size, shape, colour and general appearance.

In relation to dyspareunia and vaginismus, it provides an opportunity for cervical and vaginal visual inspection by the doctor, and gives him the opportunity to demonstrate to patient and partner what is really happening in vaginismus. The patient who has never looked directly at her genitals can be shown these by use of a simple mirror. Digital self-examination and digital partner examination can be 'permitted' under the aegis and sincere authority of 'the doctor'.

The clinical examination permits the patient who is pregnant or postpartum, who is menopausal or postoperative, who is convalescing from illness or suffering from psychological illness, for example, to ask specific questions about body and mind parts and function as the doctor is examining. This improves patient and doctor rapport, lowers patient anxiety level, and encourages reassurance from the positive statements by the doctor. It is very important to exhibit an optimistic attitude, and to avoid any expressions of hopelessness however difficult or irreversible the situation may appear at first sight. The influence of the psyche is strikingly evident in the reversal of all sexual problems. Any opening statement or look which says to the patient that it is a 'lost cause' or a doubtful cause, can prove permanently damaging. Never say 'What can you expect at your age!', however old the patient.

DIAGNOSIS AND PROGNOSIS

In general medicine, in the surgery or the outpatients clinic, after the physical examination the patient will expect you to discuss and assess your findings, make a provisional or actual diagnosis, and offer a therapeutic approach. In sexual medicine, the same postexamination pattern holds true. Perhaps in this area of dysfunction more than any other, the patient seeks not merely a diagnosis and explanation of the diagnosis but an instant solution as well. The fact that the complaint has not appeared suddenly, or the fact that it is a disturbance of a partnered act rather than a personal and individual act, fails to strike the patient as relevant to the length of time needed for control or cure. The patient wants a cure and wants it there and then. Can you give me a pill? Would hypnosis help me? Is there an operation I can have? Is there a specialist who can sort it out quickly? Would having an affair help me? Are hormones the answer? Should I come off the pill? Are injections of some kind the answer? These are typical post examination questions that the patient may throw at the doctor, even before he has written down and contemplated his findings.

The doctor must parry these questions with tact and firmness. He can do so by stating that he appreciates the patient's anxiety to get well quickly and so, between the two of them (and if appropriate the other partner), they must consider a course of action which will bring the problem under control as soon as possible. The doctor can point out that getting better needs time and effort, keenness and consideration, on the part of the patient and his counsellor. Stress again that getting better is what the consultation and any future attendances are all about, and that magic and potions are for charlatans not intelligent people. In the light of the patient's interest in getting better, the doctor can decide provisionally on a number of subsequent surgery attendances - two, three or four - which offers the patient a therapy programme without absolutely tying either side down to a deadline for a result.

STYLES OF THERAPY

For the doctor with no special training in psychotherapy or counselling skills, it may seem that tackling organic sexual problems - the smaller percentage source of sexual problems - would offer the most rewarding and least arduous area of sex therapy. In medical terms this is true, because the doctor simply applies his regular clinical skills and therapy approach, perhaps with the addition of psychological encouragement and support. Here are several examples:

(1)   Drug induced erectile dysfunction is evident. The doctor reasses the need for the drug - hypotensives, diuretics, anticholinergics - then either weans the patient off the drug or lowers the dose, or changes to a drug less likely to upset the patient. He reassures the patient and partner, and seeks a follow-up report.

(2)   The patient appears to be hypothyroid and this is primary, confirmed by T4 and TSH studies. Slow and steady replacement therapy with thyroxine commences. In monitoring patient and dosage subsequently, comment on your expectations and reassure that all body systems are recovering, including libido and outlet.

(3)   An exacerbation of osteoarthritis of hips is causing painful coitus for the middle-aged lady partner. The patient is recommended to have a warm bath or shower shortly before expected coitus, and is advised to take full dosage of analgesics not later than half an hour before coitus. She is shown alternative positions for coitus which are acceptable to both partners, is guided to use foam and supportive pillows and mattresses, or a firm base, during coitus (Table 7.1). Thought may be given on medical grounds to other help in the shape of orthopaedic referral for hip replacement, which can coincidentally improve sexual function.

(4)   A patient with mild angina is reassured that coitus is suitable with his regular partner. This applies if unhurried, if not after a meal or alcohol, if preceded by taking a β-blocker or glyceryl trinitrate, and if paced in terms of dyspnoea or chest tightness.

(5)   The patient is a male subject presenting with perineal aching, worse after coitus with discomfort and aching in the groins, and with burning or discomfort on micturition. A mid-stream specimen of urine is sent for culture to exclude urine infection. Rectal examination is carried out, revealing the boggy prostate of prostatitis. Prostate massage is followed by the prescription of tetracycline or other chemotherapy. Reassurance for quicker recovery and ease of coital discomfort is advised by temporary limiting of coital frequency, and by avoiding long periods of sitting.

(6)   Local vaginitis causing painful intercourse is reported by the lady partner. Vaginal swab taken after vaginal examination reveals the presence of candida infection, and this is treated with suitable antifungicide. Check the urine for glycosuria. Ask about any male symptoms of coital or other discomfort in case there is candida 'transfer' going on.

(7)   The patient is a diabetic on insulin for 7 years. He complains of poor erection, despite active libido and a happy relationship with his wife. Do a random blood sugar but also consider checking serum testosterone. Note urine for sugar ketones. If diabetes unstable, adjust insulin dosage. If other evidence of neuropathy - diarrhoea, paraesthesiae - consider a trial of high dose vitamins B and C such as Parentrovite. If serum testosterone is low, consider replacement therapy. Remember that bright diabetics can have psychological erectile dysfunction as well as organic, related to fear of loss of sexuality, from information read in books or passed on by fellow diabetics.

(8)   The woman has had a laparotomy for suspected peritonitis and has been left with a tender abdominal scar. She only accepts man over woman as 'normal' for intercourse. The patient is given analgesics to take before coitus. Open discussion with doctor and male partner is encouraged, to consider other coital positions that avoid pressure on the scar.

Table 7.1 Coital variations - positions for the arthritic

Male partner

(1)   Woman lying over the man: she provides most of the sexual rhythmic movements.

(2)   Woman sitting straddled over the man: same control of movements.

(3)   Side by side: man lying on his least stiff side with pillow or cushion to support still side.

(4)   Face-to-face standing position: useful if spine, hips and knees have arthritic stiffness.

(5)   Sitting in a wide chair: female partner straddled across upper legs.

Female partner

(1)   Woman lying under the man: he provides most of the sexual movements.

(2)   Man sitting straddled over woman: same control of movements.

(3)   Side by side: woman lying on her least stiff side with pillow or cushion to support stiff side - more breast foreplay possible.

(4)   Face-to-face standing position: helpful if multiple arthritic joints and if obese, too.

(5)   Sitting in a wide chair: male partner straddled across upper legs.

(6)   Vaginal intercourse with male behind her - if standing, woman can use frontal support; if lying, do so on the least stiff side.

Both partners

Be warm - take analgesics if prescribed, 1/2-1 hour, before expected coitus. Do not prolong coitus to pain or fatigue situation.

Organic causes of sexual difficulties may also require referral to other specialists for specific action. It is worth reassuring the patient or couple who have established confidence and rapport with the family doctor that they can return and talk to you after the specialist procedure. This might be, for example, treatment of cervical ulcer; repair of uterine prolapse; surgical therapy for the penile and testicular fibrosis of Peyronie's disease; stretching of a urethral stricture; removal of urethral caruncle; necessary circumcision; removal of a prolapsed disc; hip surgery; or excision of a tender episiotomy scar.

PARTNER TYPES

Before going on to look at other approaches to sex therapy, it is worth keeping in mind that conjoint interviews can give us a picture of 'partner types' which are seen to recur not infrequently. Here are four examples:

The come close - keep away partnership

One partner wants constant love and attention. The other partner needs 'space and time' alone, only occasional love and attention, freedom from any constant togetherness. In this partnership, there is a risk of sexual frustration and morbid jealousy of the partner who needs constant love, towards the other.

The I can manage - I cannot manage partnership

One partner takes on most of the weight or burden of economic, social and home activities and chores. The other partner appears inadequate, contributing but poorly to the setting, always depending on the other partner. There is a risk of the depending partner not achieving a successful sexual relationship, becoming tense, anxious or panicky at sexual advances by the other partner.

The balanced blame partnership

Both partners accuse each other of having faults that impair the relationship and disturb their social and sexual harmony. Neither partner is ever willing to admit he or she is to blame. The risk here is that first the sexual relationship breaks down, then the marriage itself falters and fails.

The worry - who cares partnership

One partner complains, worries and nags on the social and work and home behaviour of the other partner - gambles a lot, smokes too much, often drunk, frequently swearing, going off with friends. This partner, who is being complained about, listens all right but carries on behaving unchanged. The risk here is that the worrying partner develops sufficient anxiety and irritability to depress his or her libido while, by contrast, the 'who cares' partner may happily seek sexual outlet elsewhere.

These four partner types are not at all exhaustive and may be added to, with further experience in family practice and in sexual counselling. Recognition of the behaviour pattern in conjoint interview may help the doctor to guide his patient-cum-client towards insight of the pattern, and subsequently towards help in altering that pattern in a positive direction.

Individuals and couples seeking counsel or therapy are sometimes inhibited from a fuller discussion by:

Not wanting to 'shock' the doctor.

Not wanting to reveal a 'weakness' of their own or the partner.

Not wanting to 'waste' the doctor's time.

Being resentful that the partner has not accompanied the patient.

Being resentful at being pushed by the partner to attend.

Preferring to see a doctor of the same sex (this applies to men, too).

The doctor's skill may be extended if all these inhibiting factors are to be overcome, singly or in combination.

OTHER APPROACHES TO SEX COUNSELLING AND THERAPY

Listening without value judgements, commenting without destructive criticism, interpreting without being dogmatic, encouraging the partners (if both are present) to communicate without your interrupting, are useful forms of psychotherapy which can be used in many problem areas for patients. So also are offering information to fill gaps in knowledge and offering guidance to both partners in response to their request. To help define each partner's expectations and show how these may be excessive or limited; suggesting special 'homework' based on recognized techniques (or modifications of techniques) such as those of Masters or Semans or Skynner (which we shall comment upon in this book), are further areas of counselling.

The foregoing list of psychotherapeutic approaches does not come instinctively to doctors, whose role in general medicine is often paternalistic, dogmatic, evaluative, critical or informative, and leading rather than focusing. Being a listener with empathy and sympathy is a feature of good general practising in many circumstances, of couse, but being comfortable with your own sexuality, offering therapy without imposing your own moral or personal standards in sexuality, and understanding or reading the unspoken as well as the spoken in sexuality - all need additional training and skill.

Where does the interested family doctor obtain such training, raise such skills or develop these modes of therapy in sexual problems? Just as in general medicine, study of books and texts, or of articles and monographs, can provide the theoretical knowledge of sexual counselling and therapy. Skill is acquired by the daily practice of that counselling and therapy. The doctor in this area is no longer the teacher and the patient his pupil. Instead, he is a fellow traveller in the patient's problems and dysfunction, listening and looking, hearing and noting, then offering his own understanding of the material and seeing how the patient applies it.

Some doctors beginning or continuing a practice in sexual counselling prefer to act on their own initiative, developing their own style and technique in a pragmatic manner. Those who have had formal psychiatric training or training in analytical psychology or behavioural psychology may not feel the need to share their style, approach, results, difficulties and successes with fellow practitioners. Doctors, who have come to counselling via family planning clinics or antenatal and postnatal clinics or work in genitourinary medicine, may similarly be disinclined to participate in conventions, conferences or seminars which reveal their personal techniques and their outcome.

Some doctors, who are eager and determined to pursue sexual counselling and therapy, will look for more formal meetings and discussions on sexology, sexual therapy and sex counselling. This can involve attending local postgraduate lectures, advertised seminars and training courses, weekend conventions, national or international congresses on sexology, for example. Among the most significant of United Kingdom approaches to this work is that undertaken by the Institute of Psychosexual Medicine whose approach to basic training and advanced seminar development has been much influenced by the psychoanalyst, Dr. Michael Balint, and latterly by the Institute's president, Dr. Tom Main. The style of seminar training evolved helps doctors to 'become aware of their own feelings in order to understand the contribution they make to the doctor-patient relationship'. Individual patient case problems are presented by doctors attending the seminar, in order to achieve peer review and peer audit as well as to report on their own style, views, assessment and evaluations. The regular seminar discussion of ongoing cases encourages the doctor's skills and helps them to 'recognize their own behaviour patterns and blind spots' which could mar or limit successful therapy.

BARRIERS

Not every patient will require the full application of psychotherapy to help him or her achieve insight and self-modify behaviour. Some will only require straightforward explanation, clear advice, and reassurance as well as permission to act or continue in a given pathway. Some would not benefit from the listen and consider and then proceed' approach no matter how skilful the therapist physician. Significant barriers to that kind of interaction and response arise in the following circumstances:

Disturbed doctor patient communication, because of a 'foreign language barrier', or because of severe deafness, or because of religio-ethnic proscriptions.

Faulty patient reception with poor patient interpretation, because of congenital low IQ or acquired brain illness or drugs effect.

Mentally ill patients with loss of insight, that is, true psychosis.

Patients suffering from organic system disease who are too frail, too ill or too debilitated.

Patients with a good IQ but with strongly constructed self-protective barriers that do not readily permit penetration by interpreters.

The defaulting patient.

The alcoholic patient.

These categories are not mutually exclusive, and multiple elements may combine to prevent therapy for what at first sight looks 'a suitable case for treatment'.

The ability of a patient to be imaginative, that is, to manage techniques involving fantasy and fantasizing, can add to the likely success of many in the past, the daydreamer or fantasizer has been condemned as lazy or indifferent. In the field of sexuality, the male or female partner who can conjure up fantasies in their sexual activity, may not only enjoy sex more but also demonstrate to each other, for themselves, that living, loving and sexuality can be a happy and successful combination.

MIXED THERAPY APPROACH

Full psychoanalysis, along the lines developed initially by Sigmund Freud, is rarely undertaken for sexual dysfunction alone. This is because of the time-consuming and therefore often uneconomic nature of such analysis, which in any case is whole patient oriented rather than sexual dysfunction and sexual partnership oriented. The insight gained by the patient who does undergo analysis can be valuable and applied in the whole of his or her life pattern and life progress, not just confined to the sexual situation.

Behavioural psychology has certainly had much to offer the man or woman with sexual dysfunction. The non-organic disability or upset is viewed as a learned response, irrespective of the affect or personality of the patient concerned. Such learned responses can therefore be suitably modified by a variety of techniques, just as these are used in anxiety states or phobias, for example. At its most basic, the patient is instructed in specific actions, exercises or modes which offer relaxation or distraction (or both) for the pre, intra, and postsexual activity process. Where aversion is a clear contributory factor, the behaviourist can apply the techniques which desensitize or decondition and expel the aversive thinking and responses. The reader is referred to a behavioural therapy manual for more detailed explanation of such approaches as 'successive approximation', 'flooding' and 'implosion'.

Contemporary counsellors and therapists take the best of all words and utilize a mix of behavioural system, of insight guiding system, of self-assessment system, and the doctor's permission system (it is all right to do this because I know medically it is safe and sound). The therapists use this in one-to-one settings, conjoint settings and group therapy settings as seems appropriate.

TIME LIMITATION AND THERAPY

The clients of the sex counsellor, medical or otherwise, are men and women living out there in the real world of earning a livelihood, supporting a partner and self, building a home, creating a steady life

119

pattern. The time which an individual or couple is willing to give for therapy of sexual dysfunction is therefore a limited one - unless they are well-to-do enough not to care how much it costs or how long it takes to get better. This time limitation - and economic aspects - account for a higher degree of attendance fall-out than many counsellors new to the activity would have expected. A patient or couple's failure to attend, however, need not be taken as a sure sign that either all is well, or that all measures have been to no avail. The middle way is often the truth of the matter - the counsellor has been of some help and the couple or individual accepts some degree of limitation in total cure, control or recovery.

Since counsellors have to face limits on their and the patients' time, short phase therapy approaches have become the more popular therapeutic style. Such short phase counselling involves the following elements:

Lowering stress, tension and anxiety levels through words and actions, including mutual discussion, and examination plus observation.

Ensuring that all parties understand each other's needs, wants, pleasures, turn-offs, difficulties, fears and hesitations.

Determining the partner's genuine awareness and knowledge of their own and each other's sexual anatomy, and what really happens at coitus.

Outlining, drawing and explaining alternative approaches to arousal and excitation, as well as permitting the study and experimentation in other coital positionings and styles. (I call this the LEDO short phase counselling style, an obvious mnemonic of lowering, ensuring, determining and outlining.)

A FULLER HISTORY

Before we review possible therapy approaches to the many male and female problems noted in earlier sections, we should note some other relevant information and facts that we require to obtain from the attender or both partners. This will include:

Details of birth control methods - none, sterilized, vasectomy, sheath, cap, intrauterine device, hormone pills, as well as personal feelings and religious attitudes to such methods.

Details of operations - none, thoracic, limb, upper abdominal, hysterectomy, oophorectomy, prostatectomy, herniotomy, haemorr-hoidectomy, ablative lower abdominal or pelvic surgery, sympathectomy.

Details of family history - parents, grandparents, living accommodation, hierarchical roles, attitude to religion, attitude to marriage, attitude to sex.

Details of mental history - no mental illness, family mental history, depression, anxiety, attempted suicide, schizophrenia, neurosis, mania, personality disorder, mental handicap.

Details of marital relationship - first partner, second or third partner, previously engaged or betrothed, premarital sex, extramarital activities, separation, happy, stormy, placid, miserable.

The findings are noted and collated with the previously discussed 10-point questionnaire, to give the doctor a global view of the complaining patient, and the likely strong (or weak or absent) influences on his or her sexual dysfunction. The counsellor would expect a patient seeking his help to be as open, truthful, candid and straightforward as possible. This is not always the case, at least in the starting period of counsel and therapy. Lies, half-truths, omissions, distortions, misunderstandings may all be revealed if the counselling goes on. Such findings should not put the counsellor off his work - but help his assessment all the more.

The effects of drugs on libido, erection, ejaculation and orgasm have been discussed in earlier sections of this book. They show us that we must take a clear history of current, recent and previous drugs intake if we are not to overlook organic disturbance from this source - or emotional disturbance from this souce.

ADAPTABLE TECHNIQUES

Down the years, a wide range of techniques have been developed by distinguished workers in the field of sexuality - Masters and Johnson, Michael Balint, Jack Annon, John Bancroft and M.J. Crowe, for example. The widespread development of sex counselling and sex therapy has made vigorous use of whole or part of the elements of this range of programmes and regimens to help the sexually dysfunctional individual or couple. Each county, country, area, social group, has often seen local needs and conditions dictate what is used and what is set aside, what is taken directly and what is adapted. A good example of this is the technique developed by William Masters and Virginia Johnson for 'human sexual inadequacy' and known as sensate focus. This is essentially a programme for creating a new set of learned responses in the couple's sexual behaviour, whatever the individual problem, such as lack of enjoyment, poor arousal, or lowered libido.

In a sensate focus programme, as adapted from the original 2 weeks or weekend privacy in a hotel away from the regular environment, the couple are offered instructions which parallel their original courting days. Coitus is forbidden so that risk of erectile or orgasmic failure is avoided in the early programme sessions. With lowered anxiety, the couple move on to stimulating each other in a non-demanding way, clothed, then in underwear, then in the nude. They must communicate what feels good or bad, what is enjoyable or upsetting, what is positive or negative. Stroking, fondling, kissing, caressing, action and passivity give pleasure focus.

All this is non-genital stimulation. When all goes well, the next sessions permit limited mutual genital stimulation in a light and somewhat teasing approach. No response towards the orgasmic phase is asked for. For the last two sessions, the couple are guided on a suitable permitted coital position - for example, woman superior - which gives appropriate control to the non-dysfunctional partner.

In the course of sensate focus sessions from the earlier to the later ones, the couple may find a 'block' because of underlying marital disharmony or a 'delay' because of uncertainty that it 'will really work' or else the couple may find they have responded so well that, permission or not, they proceed to successful sexual intercourse. They may even fail to turn up at the next counselling session because - voila! - all is well.

The principles underlying sensate focus therapy match well with our LEDO short phase counselling approach mentioned above. Lowered stress, ensured understanding of pleasures and needs, determination of understanding sexual anatomy, and outlining the approaches to arousal and excitation, are all present within this particular regimen. The interval between such sessions - and the link with the sex counsellor - can be every few days, once a week or once a month, as convenient, but it requires a defined structure and not a haphazard format. 'Excuses' given by the individual or couple about non-activity can be taken as signals of 'the block' or 'non-acceptance' - such excuses as working overtime, never any privacy, no baby sitter, headache, felt too tired, had to finish my hobby. In such cases it may become clear that this form of behavioural approach is not going to be adequate or successful, and a switch to insight-oriented therapy is made.

THERAPY OF COMMON SEXUAL PROBLEMS

In the last part of this book, I now propose to move steadily through the common male and female sexual problems which we considered earlier, and offer a series of examples by which these may be controlled, cured or modified. This writer's views on tackling the conditions need not, of course, be considered the one and only direction or pathway in a given patient (or client, as some counsellors prefer to call the dysfunctional individual). Moreover, within the constraints of presenting material in a more precise manner, we cannot dart hither and thither tying up every loose end. The reader can consider all the aspects and conjecture whether all will be passable, well or very happy indeed, or failure looms.

REDUCED OR ABSENT LIBIDO

We noted earlier that we should separate the partner who is little interested or but rarely interested in sex yet can be aroused, from the partner who cannot be excited, stimulated or aroused in any circumstances. For the man or woman who lacks arousal but can be stimulated, possibly even to orgasm, the counsellor needs to look at the work pattern, leisure pattern, social set-up, and general sexual history of the low libido sufferer. At least two sessions, possibly more, are needed to assess preferential sexual experiences which he or she knows created sexual interest or excitement at some time in the past. These are communicated to and with the partner, who is enlisted to offer, surprise and tempt the sufferer with such 'goodies' - but not to pressurize for an immediate sexual follow-through. Where no such preferential experiences are revealed by the sufferer, the counsellor can suggest a series of sensate focus sessions along the lines noted earlier. This will open up the erotic stimuli or activity most likely to raise libido. Another approach is to give the patient permission to stop at fixed times in the day and think about (a) sexual activity and (b) his partner, imagining her with him in such an activity.

The distractions of children, parents and work may be great and not permit the intrusion of sexual thoughts in the course of the day or evening, so using the 'fixed time for thoughts' approach can cut across those distractions.

Taking a history can reveal that the low libido individual never takes a half-day or day off, never has a weekend away or a winter or summer holiday. Some 'time out' can be encouraged, even it can be pointed out, by mutually being at home for lunch but stimulating the other with sex instead. The sufferer who has been coerced to attend for counselling by the partner with an active libido, may feel resentful at being told to give up 'valuable time' to think about or take part in sexual activity. The objections are more likely to be raised by older patients or adults than by teenagers or young adults. This kind of hesitancy or objection may require a further session or sessions to permit insight orientation. It may, alternatively, cause the counsellor to lose his attender.

Lack of arousal in low libido may also indicate that the marital stability is in jeopardy because the man or woman with this state has simply 'fallen out of love' with the partner. The turn-off can be due to a whole range of factors, as we noted earlier, examples included cosmetic turn-off, boredom, age effects, change of economic or social circumstances, even the contact with new stimulating workmates or business contacts. In that case, a referral to a marriage guidance counsellor would seem useful and appropriate. When that aspect has been resolved - if divorce or separation does not ensue - then the couple can return for help in the format of the approaches mentioned above. Although short-term androgen hormone therapy has been tried for poor arousal, it is not really indicated at all unless serum studies show that the level is below normal range. A placebo response could, of course, take place.

Where the man or woman simply cannot be stimulated or excited at all, attesting to loss of libido in entirety, it requires a number of sessions to check out the following:

Any clinical illness of physical or psychological type present?

Any indications of true sexual aversion - primary or secondary?

In both cases, there is a need for an insight-oriented approach, followed by reassurance and education on risks or absence of risks. In aversion, relaxation exercise techniques as well as behavioural desensitization - in imagination or in reality, making sexual contact in successive stages increasing proximity while being reassured and assuaged by the counsellor - can be undertaken.

After a reasonable period of the short phase LEDO style approach, progress is assessed by the individual, the partner and the doctor. Absence of any progress but keenness of the couple to go on, may tempt the doctor to try - in either sex - short-term use of oral testosterone while continuing the psychotherapy, and approach of LEDO. After a further period of, say, a month, absence of any rise in libido may cause such intramarital problems that the partnership is eventually abandoned. In some cases, after that, the taking up of a new partner with dropping the old, sees the reappearance of libido with departure of the aversion.

The usual drugs history, which I have suggested is a must for all sexual problem patients, can sometimes reveal that the sex drive only began to fade when the drug therapy began to work pharmaceutically. Withdrawing the drug or lowering the dose would then reveal if the whole problem was drug induced or drug affected. Drugs may be taken by the libido-lacking partner who is trying for self-help, fearing to lose his partner because of his or her absent sex drive. Alternatively they are illicit drugs and because the partners are involved in the 'drugs scene', libido has suffered accordingly.

ERECTILE DYSFUNCTION – EMOTIONAL OR PSYCHOLOGICAL BLOCKING

In an earlier section, in Table 4.1, we systematically listed a series of patterns and sources whereby the cortical and reflex control of erection might be partially or completely inhibited. We can consider these in brief again and look at helpful approaches. In all cases, we adopt the short phase LEDO counselling approach initially, although some patients will require more sessions of psychotherapy to encourage insight and then action - as indeed may the partnering woman as well.

The 'perfect' or 'pedestal' lady influenced male erection adversely by either behaving in motherly not lover fashion, or by avoiding abandon and keeping the mood remote. Conjoint interview and free exchange of information and views might expose these patterns, permitting a look at historical sources for both partners' attitudes. Permission to 'misbehave' as well as behave, and 'let go' as well as hold on may be helpful, especially to the lady partner. A sensate focus might be added into the therapy programme as well as the use of a holiday away from the familiar environment (and familiar roles).

The controlling pseudopassive partner is another partnership member who needs separate or conjoint sessions, to help gain her confidence in sometimes being the prime mover in sexuality and not always awaiting the male partner's signals. This type of difficulty is very much helped by sensate focus sessions as well as some relaxation exercises. Sexual education in a gentle but direct manner may improve the male partner's loving and caring technique, especially if the counsellor learns what really turns the lady partner on. Again, this type of pattern often throws up a more extensive intramarital conflict which would call for referral to the marriage guidance counsellor.

The male partner who suffers from premature ejaculation, for the many possible reasons outlined in the earlier section, may benefit from a combination of psychotherapy and drugs. The psychotherapy involves lowering anxiety levels by encouraging a 'resting and relaxing' period after initial arousal. Alternatively, we may recommend the strategy of 'redirected attention', in which, at each stage of the coital programme, thoughts are concentrated on the pleasure of here and now at cerebral level - ignoring what is happening 'down below'. The self-imposed distraction should permit a longer 'holding out' of move to ejaculation and orgasm. Some doctors have combined this with occasional use of a precoital low dose tranquillizer such as Anafranil (clormipramine hydrochloride).

Two behavioural approaches are those of J.H. Semans' interrupted stimulation technique and Masters and Johnson's squeeze technique. The Semans approach is as follows. In phase one, the couple are advised to make sexual contact but to confine it to caressing and fondling, which eventually focuses on the penis. This continues until he feels ejaculation is imminent, when he at once signals the woman to stop. Once his urge to ejaculate subsides, they start again - until the next point of imminent ejaculation when he calls stop, yet again. Should he make an 'error' and come despite himself, they are reassured that it does not matter, simply start the programme again. The aim is to condition the man to longer spells before coming to orgasm. They then move to phase two, when the woman permits vaginal entrance and he can then ejaculate as he wishes. The best coital position for this procedure is 'woman facing man and lying above him'.

In Masters and Johnson's squeeze approach, the first phase is identical to Semans' technique. However, this time when the man signals that ejaculation is imminent, the woman faces the recently erect penis and places her thumb on the underside at the glans, pressing firmly with first and 2nd fingers at the side and dorsum of the penis (see Figure 7.1). This pressure is held, counting 4-5 seconds, then released for a quarter of a minute, then arousal continues till the next imminent ejaculation, when the squeeze is again applied. The partners are advised only to use the squeeze approach on a fully erect, not a floppy or poorly erect, penis. The technique is practised over five or six sessions. Again, unexpected ejaculation calls for reassurance that the programme can 'start again'.

In the second phase, the lady sits astride her partner and gives him holding confidence by using the squeeze a couple of times. At the third approach, she leans forward and places his penis into the vagina. She then moves back on the penis but does not ride the organ or move rhythmically. If he again feels about to ejaculate, she can still reapply the squeeze. In the final phase, the lady partner starts rhythmical movements and they orgasm and ejaculate at their own desired timing.

The use of local anaesthetic creams or cooling lotions has also been

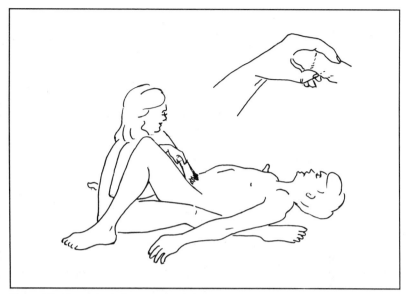

Figure 7.1 Squeeze technique - one handed

encouraged by commercial concerns. There is no proof that such agencies are anything but placebos, which are likely to fail. This refers to creams, gels or sprays, for example.

The behavioural techniques have given good results but may require continuing use over days or weeks, before being fully successful. Some counsellors have recommended the woman partner uses a simple cream on her fingers to symbolize or simulate vaginal lubrication as she applies the squeeze. The woman can use the fingers and thumb of either hand but usually does the job best with the dominant hand. The unpartnered man has little chance of using Semans' or Masters' approach very effectively, although some men claim that they have applied self-squeeze to improve erection control without premature ejaculation.

The behavioural approach should, in theory, cut across such aetiologies of premature ejaculation as guilt, fear of orifices (Freud's so-called castration complex), pedestal view of woman, and cryptic homosexuality. In practice, it may not do so and the patient will require the listening and insight-oriented approach.

We have considered the faulty function linked with either partner's birth control approach under such headings as 'blank bullets firer' and 'condom cavalier'. The various elements noted in that discussion can be brought out and offered for consideration in insight-oriented psycho-therapy sessions. Sex education on how the contraceptive approach really works, and what it directly does and does not do, can enlighten the partners and lower anxiety levels. Permission can then be given to consider alternative forms of birth control or, if the options are few, help can be given to come to terms with the situation.

Faulty erectile function linked with fear of failure can be treated by separate and conjoint sessions, using the LEDO approach. Sensate focus therapy may be helpful for the group described as easily turned off or poorly turned on. A look at the privacy or otherwise of the social setting may permit 'environs manipulation' suggestions. The couple can also be permitted to look at non-coital sexual pleasures in the process of a distraction style regimen. Orogenital sex can keep the partners interested and happy while the genital-genital situation is being treated. A more prolonged series of sessions of the 'listening and offering views' approach to psychotherapy may be required. It is important to know - and to ask gently - how much limitation of erectile capacity the man and his partner would accept, if any.

Where prolonged erectile failure occurs despite all the methods offered, the sufferer may request referral to a genitourinary surgeon for possible prosthesis. This seeking for an artificial erection by asking to consult the surgeon can be turned to good use in a psychological block. This is because the surgeon, before considering which type of penile prosthesis he might implant, will most likely check on nocturnal erections. These take place normally during sleep (during REM or rapid eye movement sleep phases) and can be picked up by penile plethysmographic apparatus. The graphs can be shown to the patient with a psychological block to help convince him, so to speak, that there is no organic defect and that reversal is still possible.

CIRCUMCISION

Two large religious groups, at least, practise removal of the foreskin of the penis in infancy or early childhood. Phimosis or other penile local problems may necessitate circumcision in later years after childhood. It has occasionally been suggested that the man with erectile failure might be directed to have a circumcision. This would expose the sensitive penile tip and 'encourage' firmer erection for partial failures. Psychological block is not, however, any less powerful in disturbing erectile function in the circumcised than in the uncircumcised. As for organic erection problems, the presence or absence of a foreskin is not at all relevant to the outcome of therapy. The only indications for circumcision from a medical aspect if required are strictly for specific organic problems, not sexual ones. On the female partner side, some women are more turned on by a circumcised penis as part of a preferential sexual experience - and vice versa. This may be a matter of visual stimulus but is occasionally related to received notions on virility or hygiene.

PHOBIAS – AND ORGANIC DISORDERS

Any of the irrational fears or phobias noted to encourage erectile dysfunction - ageing phobia, masturbation worries, genital and pelvic operations, and venereophobia - can be tackled by giving accurate, reassuring and correcting information, in the first instance. The older man or the older couple need to realize that there is no regular cut-off or fixed endpoint for sexuality in later years. The analogy of mature wine versus rough wine can help, as can stress on quality versus quantity. Nonsense notions on seminal strength can be reversed, and permission given for masturbation as often as is felt necessary. Preoperative and postoperative counselling about the operative procedures and their nil effect on sexual physiology are most important. When problems do arise, in the absence of organic effect, then the LEDO approach should benefit the man and the couple. In venereal disease phobias, the condition may become so persistent that referral for psychiatric or clinical psychological help is appropriate.

Organic disturbances, in which we have included, for practical purposes, true mental illness, have been considered in the earlier chapter. Where illness is present, the doctor must consider sexuality and sexual capacity in his helpful and positive approach to therapy for that illness. He may need to voice unspoken thoughts, and may also have to assess whether the psychological upset engendered by the illness is the more direct cause of erectile dysfunction than any organic effect.

The antisocial disturbances of organic dementia - erectile upset apart - include self-exposure, masturbation with the latter, intrusion of women's privacy inappropriately, attempts at physical intercourse, for example. Drug therapy control may be required. This can be tranquillizers like the phenothiazines. A trial of antiandrogen therapy with cyproterone acetate may prove effective and of course less sedating for the older man.

We have considered the influences on and patterns of ejaculatory dysfunction in the earlier section. These may be drug-induced or drug-influenced, and such medications can include tranquillizers, anti-depressants, hypertension controlling drugs and even the anti-cholinergic drugs. A careful drug history should reveal this aetiology and offer consideration of lowered dosage, drug withdrawal or alternative medication.

No transport of semen presenting as basent ejaculate may indeed be due to failure of semen production. This could arise in primary hypogonadism, or postinfective (viral or tuberculous) testicular disease. Orgasm may still be inact but no sperm or fructose will be present in the postorgasm urine specimen. Absence of contractile expulsion of semen can be drug-induced, may follow trauma or infection, or may derive from a neuophathy, for example. Referral for a genitourinary surgical opinion is then appropriate.

The dysfunction of achieving erection but failing to ejaculate can again be drug-induced particularly by the antidepressants. Over-controlled timing or delayed ejaculation may be the result of any or a mix of the 11 factors noted in our earlier consideration. Once again the LEDO approach may prove appropriate. Sometimes several insight-oriented sessions may be required. Discussion of alternative contraception is relevant in coitus interruptus as a source of delayed ejaculation. Cryptic homosexuality may not be revealed for many years until this appearance of retardation in ejaculation. The doctor must look for other hints of the condition before tactfully broaching the possibility. This form of disturbed ejaculation may, in addition to the topics discussed earlier, indicate a more global marital disturbance and indicate a need to refer for marriage guidance counselling. Retrograde ejaculation can sometimes respond to phenyl-propanolamine therapy or even imipramine.

THERAPY OF FEMALE PARTNER PROBLEMS

The approach for women suffering from anxiety depression or anxiety neurosis or depression is, as always, a combination of psychotherapy and tranquillizers or antidepressant medication. In severe cases, the referral to a psychiatrist is relevant. We noted earlier that depression can occur at the time of the menopause but that this is not a direct indicator for the use of hormone replacement therapy. We also saw that libido may be unchanged or even occasionally increase in depression. Non-sexual marital friction as a source of libido decline again requires referral to professional marriage guidance counselling, with or without a psychiatric assessment as well.

HORMONE REPLACEMENT THERAPY (HRT)

While sexual drive in women is not directly linked to oestrogen and progestogen, the indirect effects of decline or fall in female sex hormone levels around and beyond the menopause are well recognized.

Osteoporosis, with risk of pain and fracture, loss of skin bloom, more sagging of the breasts and skin wrinkling, atrophic vulval and vaginal changes with loss of lubricity, as well as increasing risk to coronary artery disease, are all accepted as deriving from the altered hormonal status - not to mention the hot flushes feature. When the United States gynaecologist, Robert Wilson, encouraged the use of HRT in the mid-1960s, not for short-term but for long-term usage, he had many opponents. They believed that the use of long-term HRT increases the risk of inducing carcinoma of the breast and carcinoma of the uterus in post menopausal women - or of encouraging these neoplasms when they have already begun *in situ*. Even so, some gynaecologists in the United Kingdom have permitted the use of prolonged HRT, provided the woman has regular breast checks, regular smear tests and *per vaginam* assessments, and reports any untoward health change promptly. (It is not forgotten that relatively young women, whose ovaries have been removed for non-neoplastic conditions, are given HRT.) A 6-monthly blood pressure check is also appropriate. Diabetic patients may need more observation if on insulin and HRT. Hyperthyroid states can be aggravated by HRT. The appearance of non-cyclical bleeding *per vaginam* calls for re-assessment, and evidence of endometrial dysplastic change or of mammary tumours calls for immediate cessation of HRT. The same goes for unexpected high blood pressure, uncontrolled high blood pressure, deep vein thrombosis or other thrombotic phenomena, but not necessarily for oedema or leg cramps or neuralgic headache.

The restored lubrication and healthier vaginal lining obviates one source of dyspareunia in the menopausal woman on HRT as well as offering a psychological fillip to her morale and thereby to her libido. Some workers add short-term androgens orally to augment the libido still further.

VAGINISMUS

This complaint may not only account for an unhappy sexual partnership. It may be the source of infertility even in a long time marriage, especially if non-consummation has been the souce. We have already seen that this complaint represents a vigorous involuntary muscle spasm affecting the genital musculature, effectively closing off entry to the penis when intromission is attempted. This can occur even where the relationship is a genuinely loving one or where precoital foreplay has been accepted and mutually undertaken. Analogously, the doctor who attempts to introduce a digital examination of the woman with vaginismus, initiates this response. He can therefore make the diagnosis on site. The male partner sometimes reports poor erectile dysfunction as a psychological response to the vaginismus.

The therapeutic approach is partly that of insight-oriented psychotherapy and a use of behavioural techniques.

Where a partner is available in conjoint session, the doctor can demonstrate the nature of teh complaint by encouraging self-digital examination by the woman, and digital examination by her partner. If no partner is present, the woman applies the study herself. She may dislike the idea of this self-examination and requires to be given permission with anxiety-lowering discussion, before proceeding to this deconditioning procedure. The LEDO approach helps her awareness of her own anatomy, permits an effort to assess this in the left lateral or supine position, and helps her to agree that there is no physical complaint or barrier, and that her orifice is not 'too small'.

Using the slimmest of graded vaginal dilators suitably lubricated, she is taught to insert this slowly and then deliberately tighten her vaginal muscles and then relax. Coitus is banned, as the patient is encouraged over several subsequent sessions to accept wider and wider dilators. At the widest dilator, she is invited to let her husband use his 'natural dilator' again with plenty of lubrication. The whole process is usually successful and, indeed, some couples do not wait to reach maximum vaginal dilator intromission before achieving successful coitus.

A useful modification of this approach is to ask the couple to undertake the sensate focus sessions while coitus is banned and the graded dilators are practised. This will also help the male partner overcome any erectile problems, which may have arisen in relation to the vaginismus. Sometimes the vaginismus patient is seen who has been divorced or separated from her partner, and reveals that the split has built largely on her sexual problem. Occasionally the successful therapy permits the woman to reclaim her partner - but not of course invariably.

The misunderstanding woman may offer vaginismus as 'painful or uncomfortable intercourse' but a careful history and, of course, the examination will exclude vaginismus from this group of sexual dysfunctions.

DYSPAREUNIA

A careful study of the listed causes of superficial and deep dyspareunia, noted in the earlier chapter of this book, invites us to offer our own therapy, or else refer our patient to an appropriate physician, surgeon, psychiatrist or psychologist. We should not overlook the fact that adequate correction or reversal of the organic feature - prolapse,

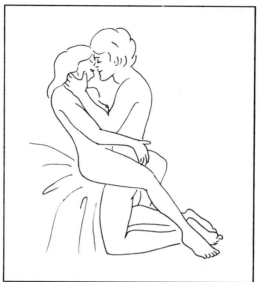

Figure 7.2 Coital position - useful in male low backache, partial erection, chronic bronchitis

caruncle, vaginitis, abscess - may yet be followed by persistence of the discomfort or pain. We are then obliged to undertake a series of 'listen and comment' sessions to determine what elements in the sexual activity, partnership and history we may have failed to (so far) acknowledge. An aversion element may be revealed and require a mix of behavioural deconditioning and psychotherapy, assuming the lady partner is willing to try. The patient is asked to write down in order of severity which aspects of sex upset her most and which aspects are least upsetting. She can then be encouraged to go through these points imaginatively, while being encouraged to relax and feel good in the session.

Low backache is due to a wide variety of factors, not all of which are amenable to therapy. Where libido is still good, the couple may require to experiment with suitable coital position for enjoying sexual intimacy. This may prove to be a standing position rather than one lying down, or else a sitting posture well propped from behind (Figure 7.2). The use of effective precoital analgesia is important in all cases. Warmth in the room and a preceding warm shower or bath are accessory helpful factors. If full coitus is just not possible guides on oral and manual loving may be offered and permitted.

SEX DRIVE STIMULATION

As an extension of the O section of LEDO, more explicit forms of sex drive stimulation have been devised and developed. These do not imply there is no need to use insight-oriented and listener therapy as well. It is simply that, using socially acceptable techniques of direct stimulation - but not surrogate partners - it is possible to raise libido levels faster and more effectively in some men and women.

The most popular form of this technique involves visual stimulation. Flat pictures, three-dimensional pictures, stills and video or movie pictures can be used. These may be classical or modern paintings and drawings, or stories of sexual activity, in which sexual organs are observed in a state of arousal, or couples are observed in sexual activity of traditional or variations on traditional patterns. Sound is excluded in this format.

The second form involves auditory stimulation. Sound films, tapes, sound videos or personal reading aloud of erotic fantasies and explicit descriptions of acceptable sexual activity can be used. Patients may recount aloud their preferential sexual experience which originally 'turned them on' in sexual drive.

The third form involves the use of non-specific relaxation instruction which precedes either of the two techniques noted above. This relaxation therapy can be practised away from the sex therapy session. Other therapists have utilized the technique of encouraging masturbation accompanied by the attachment of sexual fantasizing in a prescribed detailed manner.

ENCOURAGING ORGASM

In relation to performance anxiety, apart from insight-oriented sessions of psychotherapy, it is possible to offer the lady partner guidance on self-training to encourage orgasmic muscular contractions. In the early studies of Masters and Johnson in the 1960s, it became clear that many women failed to reach orgasm at intercourse by virtue of failed arousal. The sexual activity then becomes a sham, charade or acting procedure without the pleasure of the performance. Sex therapist Dr. P.Gillan had suggested subsequently that this orgasmic and arousal failure occurred because 'the woman has a lousy lover who lacks technique and has never even heard of the clitoris'. To be fair, the woman herself may be unaware fully of her own genital anatomy, including the site of the clitoris.

The LEDO approach can correct this lack of genital awareness. Once achieved, the lady partner can be guided in vaginal muscle training exercises, VMT for short. These exercises, still known as Kegel exercises by some, after the therapist who devised them for bladder control problems, encourage contraction and relaxation of the pubococcygeus muscle. After permission to handle the genitals has been offered, the VMT exercises can be directed in ten stages:

(1)   When seated on the toilet to micturate, spread legs as far apart as possible.

(2)   Attempt to begin, then stop, then begin, then stop, the flow of urine: this uses the pubococcygeus muscle.

(3)   Try to do these VMT exercises five times daily: within each seated session, tighten and relax ten times at 1 second intervals.

(4)   Continue with stage (3) for 1 week.

(5)   In the second week, do the VMT exercises as in week 1 but not while attempting to micturate. Double the exercises to 20 during the exercise, maintaining five sessions daily.

(6)   Continue with stage (5) for 1 week.

(7)   In the third week, do VMT exercises while thinking of sexually appealing or exciting pictures, memories, events, or people. The aim is to combine VMT with sexual fantasy.

(8)   Continue stage (7) for 1 week.

(9)   Try to increase the rapidity of contracting and relaxing the pubococcygeus muscle during the sessions so as to approximate to orgasmic 'twitching'.

(10)   In the fourth or fifth week, the woman tries her pubococcygeus contractions and relaxations at as fast a speed as she can, while accepting penis entry and holding.

This programme is flexible and there is no time limit for continuing the pubococcygeus exercises. Orgasmic experience can ensue in minor to fuller forms at any time. In the diabetic woman who complains of poor orgasmic response, the origin may be partly organic and partly psychological. A course of vaginal muscle training exercises may at least help to overcome the psychological condition by giving permission both to hope and enjoy.

PERFORMANCE ANXIETY

Where performance anxiety refers to a woman's reactions and response to her male partner's activities, then conjoint discussion becomes very important. The listening out process by the doctor can permit better communication by the partners and permit the male partner some insight to his 'turn off' actions - too rapid ejaculation, use of a condom, alcoholic odour, falling asleep after ejaculation, for example.

Performance anxiety effect on libido may be due to fear of discovery when privacy is virtually impossible. It is comparable to the sudden shut-off of micturition which a man or a woman experiences if 'caught in the act' of toilet by a stranger walking through the insecurely locked toilet door. The counselling doctor can look at possible alternatives or adjustments in environment, to help the couple overcome the problem - such as mid-day home visits, or even the use of a motel.

COSMETIC SURGERY

The problem of cosmetic turn-off - in response to ageing changes, ablative surgery, illness-induced handicap in the woman herself or in the male partner - requires a considerable talking-out and conjoint discussion process for most couples. The adaptation to altered appearance may be helped by offering the unchanged partner the following strategy:

Keep the sexual activity within as romantic an environment as possible.

Keep in mind the degree of love you have always maintained for the partner and still hold.

Concentrate on making him feel happy and wanted.

While approaching sexual contact, fantasize about your earliest pleasurable lovemaking and picture 'this is it'.

Listen to what he says about himself and reassure him of your love.

Some patients will approach the doctor about possible cosmetic surgery, for example, for face or breasts, where ageing is the turn-off. The counselling doctor needs to be clear that this is all that is wrong with the situation, and that the patient is not pinning false expectations on the corrective surgery. He may then decide that referral for cosmetic surgery is appropriate.

Even with psychotherapy and the recommendation and use of relaxation exercises, some partners are still unable to come to terms with the altered state of the disabled or changed partner appearance. The result may be formal separation or divorce or, at any rate, dissolution of the sexual relationship of the couple. Couples who have the problem of the altered partner may be helped by contact with the appropriate self-help and support group, such as the Mastectomy or Ostomy or Spastics organizations. They can offer counsel from many angles as well as the sexual one, and provide ongoing support whatever the outcome of the partners' relationship.

SEXUAL ACTIVITY AFTER AN ACUTE ILLNESS

The relevance of activity of all body systems in the four stages of coitus - cardiovascular, respiratory, muscular and genital especially - implies that any man or woman approaching sexual contact after an acute illness requires to pace out return to activity. Kissing, cuddling, stroking, touching, caressing, body contact, genital contact, intromission - this may be a useful build-up over several sessions, permitting the individual to 'pull back' if pain, dyspnoea or discomfort ensues. Exploring sessions in sex permit re-appraisal by both partners of their feelings and capacities. The following points are stressed by the counselling doctor to the patient after an acute illness:

Sexual activity should be with a regular and understanding partner.

The sessions should be in a private situation not likely to be interrupted suddenly.

The environment should be quiet and comfortable.

The session should not be undertaken after a full meal or after drinking much alcohol.

Where tablets are advised as a pre-sex aid, for example, in the use of a β-blocker in angina, these should not be omitted. Where the effects of coitus prove too strenuous or discomforting, the counselling doctor can give permission to undertake other forms of sexual relief and loving -by mutual masturbation, single partner masturbation, the use of a vibrator, for example.

As a general rule, whatever the nature of the acute illness, if the woman or man is medically fit for moderate physical activity, then that implies being well enough to re-introduce low key sexual activities described above.

HEADACHE AND SEXUAL FUNCTION

Temporary or persistent loss of libido ineither sex - but more traditionally in the female partner - may lead to avoidance of sexual contact by pleading the excuse, 'I have a headache'. The headache may be feigned or may be a genuine tension headache related to the anxiety of the sexual set-up.

The patient with true miraine (hemicrania) is unlikely to welcome sexual activity during an attack. Postural changes in coital activity may aggravate cranial blood flow changes, increasing the migrainous headache. Release of catecholamines in sexual activity can vasoconstrict vessels, further exacerbating the headache.

Apart from tension headache or migraine, the female or male partner sometimes reports headache occuring unexpectedly, and perhaps severely, during coitus. This news should not be treated lightly. It could indicate leakage into the subarachnoid space from a berry aneurysm. There could be an arteriovenous cranial anomaly which has stayed silent until this episode. Neurological opinion would seem appropriate here.

The other possibility is that this is an example of benign orgasmic cephalgia. This is a headache appearing just at or after ejaculation or orgasm. No migraine phenomena such as nausea or visual disturbance appears, although the headache is usually to one side only. Sharp or throbbing in character, the headache lasts but a few short minutes to a maximum of an hour. The headaches, having begun, reappear at each coital activity. About half of benign orgasmic cephalgia patients have a family or self-history of migraine attacks. Some patients claim the headache only occurs in 'upright' coital positions not in semi- or actual horizontal positions. Much muscular input or hurried nature of coitus increases the likelihood of such headache. Therapy requires examination, reassurance and precoital use of a β-blocker like pro-pranolol.

HONEYMOON CYSTITIS AND THE URETHRAL SYNDROME

Despite the functional interaction of genital and urinary areas in both men and women, it is usually the female partner who reports dysuria, frequency and dyspareunia after first taking up sexual intercourse - but not in every woman, of course. No gross defects of the genitourinary tract are usually observable but a bacteriuria can usually be identified. Midstream specimen of urine and swabs from the vestibule and upper vagina should reveal which organisms are present (*B. coli* or thrush, for example) and a full course of chemotherapy with coitus banned for that period should clear up the infection.

The counselling doctor should check on other relevant points:

Does the woman keep a good pre- and postcoital hygiene?

Does the woman wear tight fitting jeans or closed crotch tights?

Does the woman wear nylon, not cotton, briefs?

Does the woman fail in orgasmic lubrication - and therefore need to use a lubricant jelly at coitus?

Is the male partner a too anxious, too rapid or the non-understanding type of lover?

When all these aspects have been tackled and the infection cleared, a small percentage of women proceed to a chronic cystitis or urethral syndrome. This leads to recurring dyspareunia, suppression of libido or even sexual aversion. American surgeon, R.P. O'Donnell, claims that there are introital anatomical features which can be relevant, but unrecognized - and that careful surgery may reverse the difficulties. Mucosal and hymenal elements can produce 'valances, wattles and pressure rings' which permit local bruising and urethral meatal gaping. These can be surgically corrected in skilled hands.

Many sufferers from chronic coital-induced cystitis have taken counsel and aid from the U and I club, a self-help therapy group.

MEDICAL THERAPY FOR ERECTION

The programmes and techniques to improve libido notwithstanding, interest in a medical pharmacological approach to stimulating erection has never waned. Androgenic hormones have been the mainstay, particularly where there is implied or specific evidence of testosterone deficiency. A whole folklore of reputed erectile stimulants has come down to us through the years, including such substances as α-tocopherol (Vitamin E), procaine, the panax root ginseng, fennel seeds, mandragora, yohimbine, and rhino horn powder. α-tocopherol acts only as antioxidant in the human body and is otherwise a placebo in sexuality. Procaine has a mild stimulant effect on the pituitary-adrenal stress control system. Ginseng is considered to increase the basal metabolism slightly. Fennel seeds produce an aromatic carminative. Mandragora has a purging effect. Rhino horn powder is just difficult to obtain and is therefore likely to be an expensive placebo. The tree bark extract, yohimbine, was used in a clinical trial in 1984 by A. Morales and co-workers. Their report to the American Urological Association suggested that it was superior to placebo in organic impotence.

Direct injection of chemical agents into the corpora cavernosa of the penis to block the α-adrenoceptor flow seemed a logical approach, since α-adrenoceptor agonist therapy is one way of controlling priapism. Both phenoxybenzamine and phentolamine have been tried in this blockade but need to be carried out close to expected intercourse. Vasomotor relaxation by using intracavernous papaverine has also been used to induce erections in diabetic or arterial dysfunction. The risk is overly prolonged penile congestion. At the time of writing, these intracavernous methods offer some promise for non-psychogenic lack of erection being positively influenced by drug mechanics.

SURGICAL THERAPY FOR MALE DYSFUNCTION

Just as the surgeons may have a role to play in the organic sexual problems of women, as we have seen in organic dyspareunia aetiologies, so the erectile dysfunctions of organic origin in the male partner have been increasingly considered for surgical options. Both vascular surgeons and genitourinary surgeons have been involved in this work. In men suffering from obliterative arterial disease, non-diabetic and diabetic, the vascular inefficiency in aorto-femoral flow may present both as sciatic claudication and as an organic source of erectile dysfunction. In Europe and in the United States, vascular graft and reconstructive surgery have proved successful in arterial insufficiency. The procedures may coincidentally or deliberately improve pelvic and perineal blood flow, and thereby partially or wholly restore erectile function.

The genitourinary surgeons have evolved the penile prosthesis approach. Accepting that the handicapped of motor origin or neurological origin cannot have erection restored, implanting small plastic splints into the corpora cavernosa seemed a logical technique. Morbidity and postimplant discomfort are obviated by using an infrapubic or penile incision method. The temporarily rigid type is that, for example, of the Brantley Scott variety which utilizes an inbuilt inflation/deflation pump bulb. The permanent prosthesis is more favoured. The Jonas or Finney prosthesis is not visible at rest. The much used Small-Carrion prosthesis allows the non-erect penis to point downward, to right or left, so the patient needs no 'special' underwear. Patient and partner acceptance and satisfaction is reportedly very high.

The inflatable prosthesis has lower risk of pressure necrosis. It is useful in the paraplegic who may require to wear a sheath catheter to control incontinence of urine. Prostheses have been used in irreversible psychological impotence, under psychiatric cover.

Pre- and postimplant psychotherapy is advisable as well as conjoint counselling for the man and his lady partner, whatever the organic aetiology of the erectile problem - for emotional and marital problems may make the whole procedure pointless in the first place, or give a poor result after the event.

STUFFING' AS THERAPY

The term 'stuffing' is one of the argot descriptions of coitus. In sex therapy, however, stuffing is a technique which may be used by the partners while awaiting the male partner's implant operation, or while undergoing therapy for psychological block causing partial or complete erectile loss. In effect, the partners are given guidance to permit the man still to enjoy the sensation of 'penis within vagina'. The approach is this:

(1)   Arouse each other, until the man has his 'best possible' erection.

(2)   The penis is then gently 'stuffed' within the vagina by one or other partner.

(3)   The man relaxes, with gentle deep breaths, thinking 'how pleasant to be inside my loved one'.

(4)   He is encouraged to move his penis around, or 'up and down' while still intravaginal.

He can in reality or fantasy, picture his pleasure of sexuality and ignore the lack of full erection or ejaculation.

The co-operation of the lady partner is essential. Sometimes she indicates an aversion to the floppy or poorly erect penis. This will also require psychotherapeutic support. The principles of warmth, relaxation, privacy and unhurried approach as always apply here. The application of sensate focus therapy may also be considered alongside penis 'stuffing', so that both partners can concern themselves with mutual pleasures in an extragenital way.

CRITERIA OF SUCCESS IN SEX THERAPY

In 1980, Dr. M.F. Hussain working at the Hallamshire Hospital Psychosexual Clinic in England, suggested that the results of sex therapy could be classified under four headings of 'success'. These are:

(1)   Marked improvement - in which there is complete relief of the sexual target problem.

(2)   Improvement - in which there are substantial gains but no complete relief.

(3)   Equivocal improvement - some minimal positive change.

(4)   No improvement - no change or actual deterioration.

This approach certainly permits the doctor counselling in the surgery, in the outpatients or privately, to give some audit for the often considerable effort that he or she may put in. In this classification, there is no implication that the degree of success is likely to be permanent or likely to relapse, and it does not cover the appointment defaulters. The latter, as noted earlier, may fail to attend because of early success, dissatisfaction with the opening or subsequent interviews, marital break-up and separation, or a decision to seek the 'advice that they want to hear' from some other counsellor.

We also noted that level of intelligence is relevant. So also is intensity of purpose or determination - the 'yes', 'possibly' or 'no' answers to the question of 'do you sincerely want to improve your sexuality?' give the strongest clue to the counsellor as to when the patient or couple will attend regularly or fail to turn up. Care is also necessary in self-congratulation when success is glowingly reported. We should look again at the trigger factors or relevant agencies that sparked off the sexual problem in the first place, and see whether preventative action is needed to avoid a re-emergence of that problem later.

SEX AFTER SIXTY

In my earlier study, *Sex in Later Life,* I pointed out that ageing by itself has never been a disease. Older age is therefore not an excuse for the doctor to shrug his shoulders somewhat indifferently and make no real effort to help or counsel. Higher divorce rates notwithstanding in middle years, new marriages and remarriages continue to appear in the sixties and later. These may be solely companionate marriages or they are marriages containing some or full sexual expectations. Indeed studies on both sides of the Atlantic indicate that, in married couples over 60 years of age, coital and other forms of sexual activity are continued in just under half of all couples where the partners are able and willing. This contrasts with a figure as low as one in 20 for the unpartnered -single, separated, widowed, widowered or divorced - over sixties man or woman.

Among the regular findings which can be seen as ageing effects in the sexual aspects of a given citizen, we include the following.

For the man:

> a slowing down in speed of arousal,
> a lessened intensity of response in the vasocongestive and neuromuscular activities,
> reduced penile sensitivity,
> a lowered angle of erection of the penis,
> less semen and fluid produced at ejaculation,
> a longer time in the phase four of 'recovery' after coitus.

For the woman:

> a slowing down in the speed of arousal and greater distractibility,
> less vigour in all phases of coitus,
> reduced vulvovaginal sensitivity,
> labial and vaginal mucosal thinning,
> reduced vaginal lubricity,
> The degree and totality of such changes
> fewer or less intense orgasms - or both.

The degree and totality of such changes has no absolute in relation to chronological age.

To these basic genital organ changes, the later decades after 60 years will add a whole range of degenerative factors or specific illhealth features. These may be mild, moderate or severe and in turn may offer limitations on coital positions, effort, style and drive as for younger citizens. Because such men and women are older, the illness or disability is even more likely to create a societal assumption of negative or absent sexual feelings. Touching, kissing, caressing, never mind sexual approaches, may then be viewed askance by societal observers, who label such older citizens not as 'romantic' but as 'dirty old man or woman', not as loving and caring but as 'elderly disgusting'. In hospital, hostel, residential setting and even in the private home of relatives, no provision may be made for sexual and contact expression - rather, an unspoken ban on such behaviour tends to prevail. This bias against sexuality in later life has been prevalent not just in lay citizens but also among doctors, nurses and professional carers.

We are all familiar with the cosmetic changes of ageing. Hair greying, growing bald, wrinkling in face, neck and arms, sagging of breasts in women, paunch in men and women, stooping, slowed or stiffened joint movements, having to wear dentures or a hearing aid, are typical examples. Those age features can act as a turn-off for partner and for self. In women, dyspareunia is alleged to be more likely in the over sixties woman by reason of cumulative genital and systemic changes. This is not invariably true. There is another relevant psychosocial change seen in later life. Men seem to respond more to the club or society or organization interest in their wellbeing as well as to the caring individual. Women may consider themselves and their own wants rather than concentrating on family or husband needs or wants - and not feel guilty about it. In a sense, we see gender roles 'reversed' and this can affect sexuality.

The therapy of sexual problems in the over sixties is not unduly different from the approaches described for psychological and physical conditions in younger adults in the previous pages. The counsellor must still adopt a positive attitude and show a willingness to be supportive, empathetic and even be innovative. There will, admittedly, be more organic changes present but this should not mean abandoning the older individual or couple. Thoughtful review of the physical state, of environmental privacy, of the medication of both partners, of the understanding of sexuality by the partners - a LEDO counsel for later years - can be valuable. Helping the individual or partnership to modify or adjust their expressions of sexual loving, where appropriate, follows such a thorough review.

Because such older couples may have a greater rigidity of attitude or an undue fear of variations in sexual technique or coital positioning, for example, the doctor has to give permission as physician counsellor if such variations are deemed otherwise likely to be helpful. We have already considered the question of female and male hormone replacement therapy as possibilities and noted the risks and caveats as well as the positive side of HRT.

I began this 'understanding of sexual medicine' by suggesting that defining human sexuality is almost as difficult as defining old age. Most doctors would, I suggest, offer old age as that part of an individual human life when the adult independence of which we are often fiercely proud, moves on to a more dependent state. It may be, paradoxically, that human sexuality at all ages offers most when it lies within a context of human interdependency and is not merely standing alone.

Selected Bibliography

CHAPTER 1

Felstein, I. (1980). *Sex in Later Life*. (London : Granada)
Johnson, S. and Chopra, P. (1983). Sex myths and adolescents. *Br. J. Sex Med.*, *99*, 12-16
Riley, A. (1978). Management of sexual problems in general practice. *Br. J. Sex Med.*, *33*, 21-3
Simpson, J. L. (1976). *Disorders of Sexual Differentiation*. (New York Academic Press)
Whalen, R. E. (1966). Sexual motivation. *Psych. Rev.*, *73*, 151-63

CHAPTERS 2 and 3

Brandon, S. (1980). Range of sexual variations. In Elstein, M. (ed.) *Sexual Medicine: Clinics in Obstetrics and Gynaecology*. (London : W.B. Saunders)
Comfort, A. (1967). *The Anxiety Makers*. (London : Nelson)
Fox, C.A. (1978). Recent research in human coital physiology. *Br. J. Sex Med.*, *42*, 32-4
Jeffcoate, W.J. (1986). Impotence, science and sciencibility. *Br. Med.*, *292*, 783-4
McCrea, C. and Yaffe, M. (1981). Sexuality in the obese. *Br. J. Sex. Med.*, *69*, 24, 34 -7
Masters, W.H. and Johnson, V.E. (1966). *Human Sexual Response*. (Boston : Little Brown)
Tanner, L.A. (1978). Mythology and physiology of sexual function. *Br. J. Sex. Med.*, *39*, 35
Trimmer, E. (1977). Aetiology of obscene phone calls. *Br. J. Sex. Med.*, *21*, 37

CHAPTER 4

Berry, J. and Yorston, J. (1982). Impotence. In Draper, K. (ed.) *Practice of Psychosexual Medicine*. (London : John Libbey)
Coetzee, T. (1983). The non-reproductive consequences of vasectomy. *Br. J. Sex. Med.*, *94*, 20-5
Felstein, I. (1983). Dysfunctions - origins and therapeutic approach. In Weg, R. (ed.) *Sexuality in the Later Years*. (New York : Academic Press)

Felstein, I. (1975). Fetishism. In *Pulse* Weekly, March 22nd, 9

Felstein, I. (1982). Nymphomania. *Br. J. Sex Med., 87*, 35-6

Felstein, I. (1980). *Sex in Later Life.* (London : Granada)

Felstein, I. (1974). *Sexual Pollution: The Fall and Rise of Venereal Disease.* (London : David and Charles)

Goldstein, B. (1976). *Human Sexuality.* (New York : McGraw Hill)

Kolodny, R.C. Sexual dysfunction in diabetic females. *Diabetes, 20,* 557-9

Orner, R. and Hipwell, J. (1980). Homosexual patients in general practice. *Br. J. Sex Med., 65,* 59-61

Tomb, D.A. (1984). *Psychiatry.* 2nd Ed. (London : Williams and Wilkins)

Wade, O.L. and Beeley, L. (1976). *Adverse Reaction to Drugs.* 2nd Ed. (London : Heinemann)

Williams, M. (1977). Transvestites and transsexuals. *Br. J. Sex. Med., 26,* 20

CHAPTER 5

Blair, M. and Passmore, J. (1982). Frigid wives. In Draper, K. (ed.) *Practice of Psychosexual Medicine.* (London : John Libbey)

Duddle, M. and Brown, A.D.G. (1980). Female sexual dysfunction. In Elstein, M. (ed.) *Clinics in Obstetrics and Gynaecology : Sexual Medicine.* pp.296-308 (London: W.B. Saunders)

Felstein, I. (1972). *A Change of Face and Figure.* (London : Constable)

O'Brien, P.M.S. (1986). Premenstrual syndrome. *Br. J. Sex. Med., 13,* 78-83

Wilson, G.T. (1984). Alcohol and sexual function. *Br. J. Sex. Med., 105,* 56-8

CHAPTER 6

Dechesne, B.H.H., Pons, C. and Schellen, A.M.C.M. (1985). *Sexuality and Handicap.* (Cambridge : Woodhead-Faulkner)

Fallon, B. (1981). *Sexual Lives of Disabled People.* (West Sussex : Disabilities Study Unit)

Newman, B. (ed.) (1983). *Sex for Young People with Spina Bifida or Cerebral Palsy.* (London : Asbah)

CHAPTER 7

Crowe, M.J. (1978). The treatment of sexual dysfunction. *Br. J. Sex. Med., 43,* 22-4

Duddle, C.M. (1975). The treatment of marital psychosexual disorders. *Br. J. Psychiatry, 127,* 169-70

Felstein, I. (1980). *Sex in Later Life.* (London: Granada)

Kaplan, H.S. (1974). *The New Sex Therapy.* (London : Bailliere-Tindall)

Main, T. (1982). Seminar training. In Draper, K. (ed.) *Practice of Psychosexual Medicine.* (London: John Libbey)

Masters, W.H. and Johnson, V.E. (1970). *Human Sexual Inadequacy.* (London : Churchill Livingstone)

O'Donnell, R.P. (1978). Chronic honeymoon cystitis. *Br. J. Sex. Med., 37,* 20-3

Index of Persons

Annon, J 121
Balint, M 118
Berry, J and Yorston, J 36
Comfort, A 11
Crenshaw, RT and TL 57
Crowe, MJ 121
Deutsch, H 56
Dominian, J 83
Duddle, M 79
Fox, C 25, 26
Freud, S 119, 127
Gillan, P 134
Goldstein, B 47
Hallstrom, T 18
Hussain, MF 142
Kinsey, AC 5, 54, 79
Lee, G 101
Main, T 118
Masham, Baroness 14
Masters, W and Johnson, V 23, 25, 31, 92, 121, 126
Morales, A 140
Newman, G and Nichols, C 5
Semans, JH 126
Wilson, R, 131

Index of Subjects

AC-DC (bisexual) 53
Adolescence 2-6, 8, 11, 17-18, 50-51, 70, 76, 83, 102,127
Adultery 6, 21, 31, 41, 50, 52, 66, 83, 87, 110, 121
Ageing
  sexual changes in 5, 12, 17-18, 27, 35-41, 47-51, 65-68, 130
  cosmetic changes in 21, 41-43, 85, 89-90, 120, 136
Aggression and sex 6, 14, 17, 20, 38, 52, 56, 66, 76, 81-84, 109, 121
Alcohol and sex 40, 76-77, 83-84, 88, 96, 116, 118
Aphrodisiacs 20, 24, 52, 60, 67, 73, 77, 96, 130, 139-140
Arousal 3, 6, 15, 18-19, 23-25
Argot, sexual 12, 15, 52, 56, 109, 141
Arteriosclerosis 2, 5, 27, 32, 45, 58, 65-67, 72, 129, 142
Autonomic control 23-25, 32, 43, 45, 47, 63-65, 74
Aversion, sexual 9, 58-59, 120, 129

Bartholin's glands 24, 85
Behaviour, sexual 1-4, 6, 9, 11-16, 18-22, 38-49, 52-57, 70-77, 85-92, 101-103
Birth control
  see Contraception
Bisexuality 3, 53-54
Blood pressure in sexual response 24-26
Breasts
  ageing changes 3, 17, 92, 136
  in sexual response 13, 24-25, 41, 60, 100
  mastectomy 45, 90, 99, 120
Buggery 12-14, 54, 76, 83
Bulbo; cavernosus muscle 25, 46, 68

Chronic illness
  effects on sexuality 19, 42, 44-46, 48, 64-70, 73-75, 81, 85, 97-99, 138
  coital positions and 28-30, 133
Chromosomes 2, 3
Circumcision 128-129
Climacteric
  female 2, 18, 50, 81-82
  male 2, 19, 50
Clitoris 28, 85
Coitus
  age aspects 19, 93, 99, 111, 140, 143
  definition in phases 24-26
  disorders and dysfunction 27, 32-33, 35-43, 52-57, 58-70, 87-97
  drugs and 73-76, 95-97
  interruptus 40, 47, 48, 86, 130
  painful 70, 84-86, 93-95, 113, 133
  positions and 27-30, 114, 125-127, 133
  pregnancy and 30, 86
  privacy and 39, 47-48, 101, 125
Contraception 2, 37, 39-40, 75, 86, 88
Counselling 7-8, 37, 57, 103, 112, 117-128, 129-135
Cosmetic surgery 136, 140
Cunnilingus 14
Cyproterone acetate (anti-androgen) 73, 129
Cystitis 85, 138-139

Dementia 66, 72-73
Depression 17, 37, 44, 71-72, 77, 81-82, 90
Diabetes mellitus 19, 21, 45, 48, 63-64, 81, 98, 114, 131, 140
Drugs and sexuality
  positive effects, 32, 36,53, 65, 85, 113, 130-131, 139-140

negative 36, 44, 46, 73-77, 95
Dyspareunia 18, 41, 84-94, 113, 131-
133, 138, 143

Education, sex 1, 5-7, 18, 20, 43, 54,
102, 105, 110, 117, 122
Ejaculation
presentation and problems 9, 11-14,
17, 24-26, 37, 45-49, 126
the phases of 45
Environment and sex 20-22, 26, 39,
55, 88, 122, 143
Erection, 6, 12, 23-26, 31-33
- dysfunctional 35-41, 44-45, 50-
51, 63-69, 72-78
Erotic stimuli 4, 6, 13, 15, 20, 24,
110, 120, 125-126
Excitement phase of coitus 23-25
Exhibitionism 15, 66, 76, 90
Experts, sex 3, 7, 31

Fantasising 6, 13, 24, 40, 47, 59, 124,
134, 135
Fashion and sex 2, 6, 18-19, 21, 101
Fear and sexuality 8, 15, 19, 37-44,
50, 55, 64, 66, 71, 81, 83-89
Fellatio 12, 14
Fetishism 60-61
Foreplay 6, 13, 24, 28, 38, 42, 55,
58, 60,
88, 103, 126
Frigidity (now called
altered female libido), 58, 81-
86

Gay 6, 53-57
Gender orientation 3-5
General practice
counselling in 7-8
sexuality problems
presenting in 4, 7-9, 19, 29-30,
57, 59, 82, 97, 100, 107-113,
116-120, 131, 137, 144
Genital organs
awareness 6, 8, 85, 120, 141
responses 25-27, 32, 36-37, 81, 88,
93-94
Gonorrhoea 18, 45, 68, 87
Guilt feelings 6, 15, 37-41, 51, 91,
121
Gynaecomastia 74, 75, 76

Hair
sexual 3, 15, 24, 41, 60, 65
tonsorial or scalp 41, 89, 144
white or grey 37, 144
Headache, sexual 85, 92, 138

Hearing and sex 6, 14, 24, 101-103,
116
Heart or coronary disease 19, 42, 45,
75, 90, 113, 131, 137
Heredity 3-4, 54-56
Hermaphrodite 3, 51, 53
Heterosexuality 6, 9, 13, 23
Homosexuality 3, 6, 13, 18, 48, 53-57
Hormones
female sex 3, 18, 21, 59, 75-76, 80,
92-97, 120, 130, 143
male sex 3, 4, 17, 18, 23, 24, 45,
48, 62,65, 70, 80, 99, 114, 139
pituitary 3, 24, 45, 51, 64, 75, 99
thyroid 24, 45, 63, 93, 99
HRT (replacement therapy) 96, 130-
131, 144
Hygiene 22, 41
Hypersexuality 52-53

Impotence
see Erection,
dysfunctional
Incest 14
Intercourse, sexual *see*
Coitus
Infectious diseases *see*
Organic, illness or Venereal
diseases
Insulin 49, 63, 64

Joint counselling
(co-therapy) 30-31
Joint disease and arthritis 19, 21, 27,
45, 69-70, 85, 99, 102, 113-
114, 133

Kegel exercises 135
Klinefelter's disease 4

Labia 25
Language of sex
see Argot, sexual
Lesbianism
see Homosexuality
Levodopa 32, 66-68
LEDO 120, 122, 124, 125, 128-130,
132
Libido 5, 44, 49-53, 63, 67, 71, 73,
77, 79-82, 84 85, 89-91, 96-
100, 123-125
Love 19, 22, 42, 115, 124

Marriage
and sex 2, 5, 6, 15-18, 41-42, 50,
55-61, 82-86, 89, 91, 104, 121,
142

partner types   115-116
Masculinity   3, 4, 17, 29, 39-40, 54,
      65
Masochism   14, 61
Masters and Johnson
      techniques   31, 117, 126
Masturbation   5, 11-13, 43, 66, 69,
      103, 129, 137
Mechanical problems   9, 21, 28, 45,
      63, 66, 70, 85, 88, 97-100, 101-
      105, 224, 126, 142-143
Menopause   18, 50, 79, 80-85, 92-95,.
      110, 111, 130-131
Menstruation   3, 75, 80, 87
    - and PMT   92-97
Middle age   2, 18, 21, 27, 48, 50, 62,
      63, 69, 76, 82, 89, 92, 113

Nervous system
      disease effects   37, 44-48, 63, 64, 67-
      68, 96, 102-105
      in sexual function   21-26, 31-32
Nipples   24, 28, 60, 76
Nymphomania   52-53

Obesity   20-22, 29, 41, 89
Oestrogen   18, 59, 75, 96, 130
Oro-genital sex   12, 40, 55, 103, 105,
      128, 137
Organ size, penile   50-51
Orgasm
      dysfunction   11-14, 32, 36-39, 44-
      51, 64, 69, 74, 87-89, 95
      physiology   25-28
      therapy   104, 134-135
Osteo-arthritis
      see Joint diseases
    - ostomy operations   37, 41, 68, 90,
      97, 121

Paedophilia or pederasty   14, 57, 84
Pain and sex
      see Dyspareunia,
      Masochism, Sadism
Parkinsonism   32, 37, 66-67, 76
Partner surrogates   31
Partner types   115-116, 136
Penile prosthesis   128, 140-141
Penile substitute or dildo   13
Penis   3, 13-15, 24-27, 32, 49, 59, 62,
      66, 141, 143
Performance, sexual   9, 19, 37, 40, 64,
      134-136, 142
Peyronie's disease   35, 62, 115
Perversion   6, 17, 20, 88
Phobias   42-44, 58, 84, 129
Pill, the   96-97

Plateau phase   25
Pornography   6, 88, 120
Positions *see* Coitus
Postnatal state   100-101
Preferential sexual
      experience   6, 17, 55, 120, 123
Pregnancy   28, 80, 86, 91-92
Premature ejaculation
      see Ejaculation
Premenstrual syndrome
      (PMT)   80, 92-93
Priapism, partial   26, 74
Privacy and sex   21, 101, 122, 123,
      136-137
Prolactin   75
Prostate   43, 45, 49, 62, 76
Prostitution   16-17
Psychotherapy   7, 44, 48, 70, 112,
      117, 119, 120, 125-127
Puberty   3, 5
Pubo-coccygeus muscle
      (VMT),   135

Rape   6, 14, 76, 83-84, 121
Rapid eye movements
      (REM sleep)   32, 128
Rectum   12, 13, 14
Redirected attention   119, 122, 126
Reinforcement   4, 6, 48
Religion   2, 6, 8, 90-91
Renal failure, chronic   70
Reproductive system   12, 23
Retarded ejaculation
      see Ejaculation
Retrograde ejaculation
      see Ejaculation
Rheumatic diseases   70, 113-114

Sadism   3, 14
Satyriasis
      see Hypersexuality
Schizophrenia   37, 52, 90
Scrotum   12, 25
Self-esteem and
      understanding   5, 17, 18, 21,
      40-47, 51, 55, 59, 83
Semans technique   127
Semen   23-25, 45, 48, 49, 130
Sensate focus   122-127
Sex assignment and
      chromosomes   3
Sex aversion   41, 43, 50-52, 58-59
Sex, extra-marital   41, 52
Sexual behaviour   3, 9, 11-22, 104
Sexual intercourse
      see Coitus

Sexual turn-offs   30, 35-41, 73-77, 88, 92

Sexual turn-ons   21, 24, 28, 92, 120, 139

Sexual responses   2, 14, 15, 18, 24-26, 88, 93, 109

Sheath (condom)   39-40, 86, 88

Sleep   32, 89

Sperm *see* Semen

Spinal cord   46, 67

Squeeze techniques   125-127

Stuffing   141

Surgery   99, 114-115

Swopping   61

Syphilis   68, 87

Sugar diabetes
     see   Diabetes mellitus

Technique, sexual   6, 11-14, 18, 27-29, 41, 47, 124, 134, 136
     see also Masters and Johnson, Seman, LEDO, Kegel techniques

Telephone and sex
     see Obscene telephone calls

Temperature   24-26

Testes   25, 26, 65
   - and orchitis   45, 48, 62

Testosterone   3, 4, 24, 65, 124, 139

Thyroid hormone
     see Hormones

Touch and sex   6, 24, 59, 102, 122

Trans-sexualism   59

Transvestism   60

Turn-offs/Turn-ons
     see Sexual Turn-offs/ Turn-ons

Turner's syndrome   4

Unlawful sex   14, 20, 52, 72, 83

Urethritis   46, 62, 63, 64, 81, 98

Uterus   24-26
   - and hysterectomy   99

Vagina
   infection in   57, 62, 68, 85, 87, 94, 138
   lubrication of   25, 27, 64, 75, 80, 85, 90, 95, 109, 113, 130
   sexual response in   6, 13, 18, 20, 23-26, 71-72, 85, 90, 98, 131, 143

Vaginal muscle training (VMT)   135

Vaginismus   3, 9, 18, 39, 58, 81, 93-94, 109, 111, 118-119, 129, 131

Vasectomy   37, 39, 48

Venereal diseases (including AIDS infection)   1, 7, 41, 44, 62, 68, 87, 94, 95, 113

Venerophobia   40, 44, 87, 129

Videos   15, 20, 134

Vibrator   137

Voyeurism   12, 51, 72

Women's liberation   18, 56, 79